The Real You is Skinny

Alyssa M. Dahl

Praise from readers who needed inspiration …

"Reading this was like a weight off my chest"

Megan, Canada

"Finally someone put into words how I have been feeling"

Johanna, Hungary

"Everything … just makes perfect sense"

Julie, Australia

"Changed my outlook on life … I am so motivated its crazy"

Eliza, Florida

"Motivated me to make a change to my life forever so I can be the person I want to be"

Lindsey, New York

"I just signed up for a 5K, and I am one of those people who hates to run … wow … tears in my eyes"

Kate, New Mexico

"Made me absolutely lose it crying … words will never be able to sum up how thankful I am"

Jane, England

"Knocked me right off my feet … so inspiring"

Jenna, California

"Seriously changed who I am"

Courtenay, Michigan

"I've been learning English for eight years, but it had never been really useful. Until now."

Corinna, Romania

. . . and from some who needed more

"I'm abandoning the starving and the tears and the fasting"

McKenzie, Ohio

"Literally my inspiration to throw my anorexic tendencies out the window"

Ashley, California

"I'm bulimic and have been for a year. I've been getting help from my doctor, but it's not that useful ... thank you from the bottom of my heart for inspiring me to stop bingeing and purging ... you've saved me from the worst thing in my life"

Sierra, Colorado

"Inspired me to shed my unhealthy and destructive behaviors and attitudes towards weight loss ... I've not only seen a change in my body, but I am now also in a better place mentally, and for the first time in years I can truly say I am totally content with my life"

Natalie, England

"Thank you for giving me hope that I really can become the healthy, happy person I've been trying to find for what seems like forever now"

Emily, Texas

All things reported in this book actually happened.
However, certain facts have been changed or omitted
to preserve the privacy of those involved.

ISBN: 978-1-48-495720-2

Except where noted, all advice in this book is based entirely on the
opinions and experiences of the author, who lacks professional ac-
creditation in medicine, psychotherapy, and athletic training.
Consulting with your physician is recommended before attempting
to lose weight.

Links to third party websites are provided by the author in good
faith and for information only. The author disclaims any responsi-
bility for the materials contained in any third party website referenced in this work.

Acknowledgments

I thank God that I found the online weight loss community, because it opened my eyes, put wind in my sails, and gave me life.

I thank the people closest to me who always had a kind word when they saw me struggling, who never failed to compliment me each time they noticed I was slimmer, and who often ate better around me to make my life easier.

I thank my online friends who cheered me in my successes, sympathized with me in my failures, and supercharged my spirit with their never-ending loveliness.

I thank my test readers Juliette L., Joanna C., Aimee C., and Victoria C. for helping make this book half as irritating as it formerly was, and my secret model and photographer who had the same effect on the book's cover.

Tomorrow never comes. Choose skinny today.

Contents

Preface *ix*
Introduction *xi*

1. From Fat and Awkward to Skinny and Confident *1*
2. Peak of Summer, Peak of Weight *13*
3. Questionable Methods *23*
4. Getting Smarter, Getting Skinnier *27*
5. How Much Food are We Talking Here? *39*
6. On My Way Down *47*
7. Exercise *67*
8. Learning to Fly *75*
9. On Eating Disorders *93*
10. Hitting My Stride *101*
11. Making it through Cravings and Plateaus *117*
12. My Last Year of Being Fat *123*
13. Motivation and Giving up *137*
14. A New Year, a New Me (Right?) *143*
15. How Skinny is Skinny Enough? *157*
16. More Tortoise than Hare *161*
17. When Others Get You Down *169*
18. "Springing" Back *175*
19. Is This the Moment? *181*
20. Finding Motivation When You're Almost There *187*
21. Summer of Skinny *193*
22. Surf Lessons *205*

A: Nothing Fits! *215*
B: How to Run *221*
C: Food and Drink *227*
D: The 1200-Calorie Myth *239*
E: Hating More than Just the Fat *245*
F: Complaint Department / Is Big Beautiful? *251*

Is Skinny a Valid Goal, Revisited *265*

Read This if You're Tired of Being Fat

Hello, my sweet friend. I am sorry you are in so much distress. I know how much it hurts.

The best part is, you are ready to deal with it.

But before we go any further, there is one thing you must know: if you want to succeed, there is only one way to do it. You must decide that this is going to be a permanent change. If you are looking for a quick fix, or only want to work at it for a while and then go back to your old ways, you are going to be a very unhappy person because you will eventually wind up undoing all of your hard work and hating yourself. Some people can eat whatever they want; others like us must realize that eating is a necessary evil. Eating just for fun? Not anymore; not unless you want to stay fat. If you are willing to give up the temporary comfort, the short-term pleasure, the destructive use of food as self-medication for depression, anxiety, anger, and whatever else ails you, then you are ready. You are ready to be skinny.[1]

It is going to take too long. It is going to be too hard. You are going to alternate between exhilaration and frustration, between cheering and crying. But you know what? Before long, a month will have passed. A month of hard frigging work, where sometimes even the hours and minutes take forever because you just want to stuff your face so badly—but still you fight it. And it's still just so damned hard. But after that month has passed, you will be skinnier. You will be so very happy about it. You will want to keep going. And you will.

And, unfortunately, it will stay hard. Only it won't be as hard as it was at first, because your body is getting used to this and learning who's in charge. You will keep it up, and you will start to love the new you.

But then a day will come when you look at how far you've come compared to how far you still have to go, and you will just want to collapse, because it seems like you are so far away from your goal that you'll never get there. So you'll ask your-

---

[1] By "skinny" I mean "without excess fat," not "so thin it's unhealthy."

self, "*What are my options? Give in, eat a giant burger* (which you won't even enjoy anymore) *and go back to my old ways, or keep on running this race no matter how much I can hardly stand it?*" You will realize that you can never again embrace the old way, because it is a dark, dark, lonely place full of despair. You will keep on trying, even though it seems like you will never win. Because you must.

And, before you know it, more time will have passed. But you will be so much happier with your new self that you won't believe that so much time has elapsed and so many pounds have evaporated. All the agonizing you did, all the restraining yourself when you so badly wanted just to give in … it will all seem like so long ago, like such a small thing. Just a vapor in the memory of your past. You will wonder why you ever wanted all that food in the first place.

Then, you will begin to realize that suddenly it's not such a burden anymore. It feels natural. You won't be craving those burgers and fries and pizzas because you're simply not even into those things anymore. You're just *over* them. You will wonder why on Earth it took you so long to realize this. You will ask yourself, "*Why did I ever wait so long to set myself straight? I could have done this ages ago!*" And instead of having to try to talk yourself into eating well each day, you will find it's actually hard to want to eat poorly because that just flies in the face of all you've done and who you've become.

And you will wonder what happened to you. You will think, "*I'm just a big, ugly loser, because that's simply who I am, right?*" But you'll look in the mirror and that's not who you'll see. Because you won't be that person. You'll be the real you. The lovely you. The slender you. The you who has broken free from the chains with which you formerly bound yourself and who has healed from the wounds you formerly inflicted upon yourself. You will be beautiful. You will actually begin to like who you are. You will cry from relief. You will cry with gratitude. You will cry because you don't even know what you feel, it's all so new and overwhelming.

What you will be experiencing, in fact, is new life.

What is This Book?

This book is, I hope, the answer you've been looking for. It's for people who have tried to lose the weight but believe they never can. It's a way to learn to enjoy being in your own body. And it's a true account of one girl's finding victory and freedom.

At first, this was just my story. Then, after I started sharing my story online, I got a bewilderingly large amount of feedback from people who had taken my story and turned it into *their* story. Some of these brave souls saw reflections of themselves in my depiction of who I used to be—and realized that they no longer had to be that person. Others were former prisoners to the demons of eating disorders who recognized the free person they wanted to become, and realized they needn't remain hostages to their own minds. Some were even attractive fit people who happened to be tiring of the struggle required to stay that way, and who needed a little something to keep them going.

Whichever you are, I invite you: join us and create *your* story. Come along with me and learn how to overcome the crazy thoughts and how to navigate the treacherous waters we must traverse to reach thinner shores, while fending off the rivals who seek to lure us off course.

Although this book is filled with advice on eating, exercise, and forming good habits, it is *not* a "diet," a cookbook, a trendy workout, or mere words of feel-good puffery. There's already too much tired, oversold, confusing, irritating, contradictory, cliché, and just utterly crap advice out there. Advice on "revving up" your metabolism, "targeting" fat loss in certain parts of your body, gorging on foods that "actually make you lose weight!," and constant "Top Ten" lists of odd things you can do to burn excess fat. By the way, how *has* all that advice been working for you lately? Exactly. You don't need more of that.

Instead, you will find here advice that works, presented in a way you have never seen. You'll see no 30-day, 60-day, or whatever-the-flavor-of-the-week is workout which will at first work wonders but quickly bore you to tears. You'll find no one-size-fits-all mentality, nor any fantasy method to somehow "trick" your body into forgetting what you stuffed into it last night. Your body is *your body*, and this book will help you figure out what it takes to get your body into the shape you want it to be.

Also—and this is what others have found to be the most important thing—you will find the story of someone who started out hating being fat and wishing desperately for *anything* that would provide her freedom from that misery, but who one day found herself slender, bewildered by a life filled with unpredictably wonderful experiences.

Are you ready?

(Yes, you are)

1 | From Fat and Awkward to Skinny and Confident

Forget where you've been.
Ignore where you are.
Focus on where you want to be.

This chapter is the short version of the story of how I lost the weight. For some reason, it has changed lives. Of everything I've ever written, it is the one thing which has produced the greatest number of joyful and tearful responses. I figured I'd better share it with you right up front. It has six parts.

1. Life, trapped in fat
2. The day it all changed
3. New eating strategies
4. Putting feet to plans
5. The requisite change
6. Picking up the pieces
7. (There's actually a seventh, hidden at the end of the book)

HISTORY (BEFORE FREEDOM, BEFORE SUCCESS)

I have been fat all my life. It's part of my identity. Even when I was little (if that's the word), I was roly-poly, and the other kids were faithful to remind me about it. My highest weight was 171 pounds (not insanely heavy, but it was *very* noticeable on my slight 5' 7" frame). That was several years ago. I lost a lot of that weight and got down to a respectable weight (but still flabby at 132 pounds) over the course of about two years of regular exercise and avoidance of large meals. Then my situation changed, and for some reason, I stopped losing weight, then slowly began gaining it back. I didn't notice much of a change in my habits (other than starting to drive more often, rather than walking), but I did notice a change in the fit of my clothes. Somewhere along the line, I slowly lost control of my eating.

Over a period of three years, my weight crept back up, and up, and up, all the way to 167. I simply had no idea how it was happening! I didn't think I was eating very much. I kept thinking that my weight was going to go down any day now. It didn't. I just got fatter and fatter. I felt completely helpless. I didn't know what to do. I tried to eat better and to exercise, but I failed at both. I took a class in behavior modification and as my term project created a detailed plan of how I was going to lose weight. I got an "A" in the class. I also kept getting fatter.

Then, one day, everything changed. That was the day I discovered thinspo.

CHANGES (OMG, I CAN DO THIS?!?)

Well do I remember the moment I first found thinspo. I felt like I had stuck my finger into the electric socket of inspiration. Searching online for "before & after" weight loss pictures, hoping that I would be spurred on by seeing how much better others looked after they got in shape, I stumbled upon the world of thinspiration.[2] Girls would post page after page of pictures of beautiful bodies. There were flat tummies everywhere. Collarbones. Hipbones. Elegant necks sloping into delicate shoulders. Even tons of girls looking simply amazing in nothing more exotic than jeans and a sweater, because their clothes just looked so perfect hanging from their slender bodies. It made me want that kind of beauty.

But wanting wasn't enough; I'd wanted that all my life. What gave the strength to change, oddly, was seeing how often these skinny girls were complaining about how hungry they were, how disgusted they were with themselves after they ate too much, and how little they felt like exercising. Of course, some took it too far. Many obviously had EDs.[3] I cried inside when I saw one write, "This isn't working rapidly enough. Starting today, I'm going to fast for as long as I can." She never posted anything again. However, for some reason, seeing all

---

[2] Thinspiration, also known as thinspo, is pictures of slender women (for example, the cover of this book) and stories of weight loss. The pictures inspire you to achieve slender beauty. The stories remind you that it's possible.

[3] Eating disorders.

this pain in her and others flicked a switch in me. I saw what I had been lacking all my life.

I had always assumed skinny people were skinny because, for them, it was easy to stay slim. I blamed my fatness on my slow metabolism and my lack of willpower. I figured that other people could lose weight, but I never would. I was just not strong enough. When I saw instead that tons of girls were making it happen by losing the weight, and that it was *HARD* for them, *it was a gigantic revelation!* Just HUGE! When I saw that it was hard for others, but they still struggled through it until they found victory, I thought, "*Hey, it's HARD for me, too! But hard isn't the same as IMPOSSIBLE, is it? And if it's hard for others, but they still succeed, maybe I can succeed!*" This marked the beginning of a new era.

Newly armed with the knowledge that this was going to be tough, and ready to do battle, I decided to go to war. I drastically reduced my portions from over 2000 calories per day (they just added up so fast!) to well under 1000. For the first couple of weeks, I can't lie, *it was a real bitch.* But since I knew to expect it to be HARD, instead of *whining*, I *REJOICED!* I felt a euphoric sense of *accomplishment.* When I felt hungry, instead of freaking out and dropping everything until I located food, I just smiled to myself—because I knew my hunger was making me skinny. *I was finally, for the first time in my life, really in control.* I was making good choices and reaping the rewards. I instantly started shedding weight and feeling on top of the world. Hungry like a beast at times, but on top of the world nevertheless.

Here's what my journey looked like:

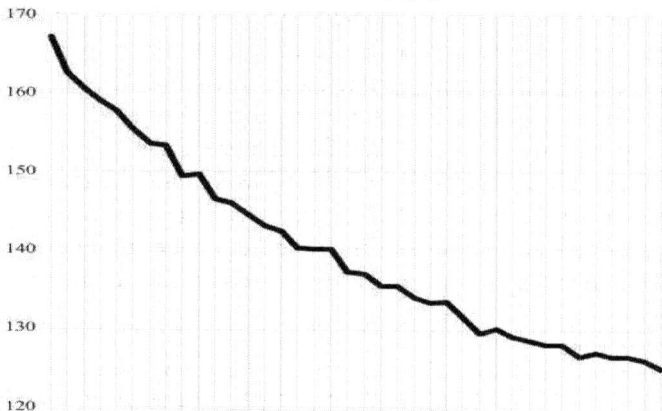

Major weight came off straight from the beginning, including four pounds my first week. I quickly lost some puffiness in my face, and I immediately felt extra room in my jeans. Within a couple of weeks, even friends started to notice, which was such a high! It was all extremely hard at first, but after a matter of only a few weeks, it ceased to totally suck. From there, I simply never stopped.

As you can see from the graph, the weight loss slowed considerably as I neared my goal, and there were several places where I hit plateaus for weeks at a time. But I made it. I actually made it! And, although the graph ends at 125 pounds, which was my goal, I didn't stop there.

EATING: HOW MUCH, HOW OFTEN?

The key to my success has been for me to keep my mouth shut. This is the most unnatural-feeling thing in the world. What do you do when you're hungry? You eat, right? Yes, you do, and that's why you're fat. Once I learned that *hunger is not always a sign that you need to eat, but it's sometimes a sign that your body is a whiney bitch*, I finally found freedom.[4]

I don't mean to say that I starved myself. Starving yourself is crap. It does more harm than good. What I did was simply WAIT before feeding myself, and when I did eat, I ate only a little, just enough to make the hunger go away. It totally worked. This was my first big lesson in thin: hunger can actually be a GOOD thing! It means you're not eating more than you need.

When I first started, I began by eating fairly tiny meals. Hunger would come pounding on my door like it was some kind of heinous emergency. It wasn't. I would ignore my hunger. In fact, I would even mock it. *"Oh, you're hungry are you? Well stuff it, fat body! You deserve to be hungry!"* The best thing was, *the hunger would always go away.* I was so elated! I realized that *hunger isn't always real!* Or at least hunger isn't nearly as serious as it would have you believe. It can be put on hold.

Of course, hunger will always return. At that time, you have the choice to ignore it again or deal with it. I tried to ignore it, and it still usually went away. However, if I was starting

---

[4] If you find yourself thinking this book encourages EDs, please reconsider. Soon, I will address all your concerns.

to really feel hungry, I didn't want to be foolish about things and develop an ED, so I would eat—only NOT a full meal! I would eat only a little, perhaps 100 – 200 calories. *Guess what? The hunger would subside every time!* When the hunger later returned, I would repeat the cycle. In this manner I managed to come into CONTROL of what I ate. And the pounds just fell off of me.

It gets even better. After a few weeks of eating like this (believe me, it was a huge battle—this crap was, as I stated previously, *HARD*—but I was just so *OVER* being fat that I chose to not give up nor give in, as I *had* to see if I could really make it work this time), *I noticed something wonderful. I wasn't hungry anymore!* I mean, seriously, even eating tiny portions, I ceased to be hungry! *I actually trained my body to get by on less food.* I "shrank my stomach"! I was a gigantic step closer to being a new person.

I don't want you to miss this, so I'm going to say it again: *it became EASY to eat well!* After a few months, it even came to feel *natural.* Again, let me remind you that I have gone my whole life without any kind of willpower, but it still became EASY for me to eat tiny portions! If I can do it—and I was a lifelong failure—anybody can do it.

Here's the best part. After I made it through this "Boot Camp" season (if I may so liken it), and healthy eating became a *habit,* I no longer needed to be so severe. That whole "no eating when hungry but waiting until REALLY hungry" attitude was important when first starting out, because I needed to teach my stomach that I was no longer its slave. But when I got to the place where I stopped being hungry all the time (remember, this took weeks!), I was able to ease up on myself. This is because after I got used to getting by on little, I tended to not become hungry until I actually *did* need to eat something. *Isn't this awesome?* I resumed being able to eat *whenever I felt hungry* (BUT, of course, only a little at a time)! This was a huge improvement from having to forcibly beat my hunger into submission all day long.

Now, before getting into how much daily food intake was involved here, I need to make sure you understand one important *caveat.* I'm convinced that the *only reason* any of this became easy for me is because I *never* binged. Bingeing stretches your stomach (or at least your appetite) back to its former (way too huge) size, and you have to start all over again. It doesn't make things impossible, but it does increase the length of time you have to keep putting yourself through this crap. Just like nobody would sign up for the army if their entire career was to be one long Boot Camp, you don't want your entire weight loss experience to be as tough as it is in the beginning, or you will soon want to give up. Please, trust me: just tough it out, DO NOT let yourself binge, and you WILL shrink your stomach, after which time it will become EASY for you to get by with less food. After that, the pounds will take care of themselves. This isn't just my opinion; scientific research agrees. Hang in there, and you *will* succeed!

Okay now, let's talk food. You might want to know *how much* I ate. I aimed for below 1000 calories per day. Calm down, I didn't say I *ate* that little, I said I *aimed* for it. However, like most people do, I pretty much always exceeded my goal. Had I actually aimed for, say, 1200 calories, I don't even want to think about how much I would have eaten, nor how fat I would still be. But by aiming for less, I wound up eating closer to 800 or 900 calories, and almost never exceeded 1200 in a day. Let me tell you, 1200 calories came to feel like a *lot* of food. Seriously, I virtually re-wired my brain so I simply no longer *need* to eat nearly as much! Forgive the cliché, but this isn't a *diet*, it's a *lifestyle*. A healthy, livable lifestyle.

Let's step back for a moment. I know what you might be thinking. Because the "official" medical professionals' recommendation is 1200 calories per day for women trying to lose weight, many people feel it is a grave sin to dip below that number. Well guess what? Medical professionals also created the special "VLCD" (Very Low-Calorie Diet) which feeds an 800-calorie-per-day diet to MEN(!) who need to lose a lot of weight, and the men don't keel over dead.

Naturally, this isn't 800 calories of french fries washed down with sodas; what makes the above-mentioned program special is that it's supervised by doctors in order to make sure patients get all their vital nutrients. The point is, if *men* can be fine at 800 calories, there seems to be no reason why *women* who meet all our nutritional needs with natural, nutrient-dense foods can't be fine with the same number of calories.[5]

Anyway, that's enough talk about food for now. We'll talk

---

[5] For more on this, including proof that eating this little can actually be better for you, skip to Appendix D, "The 1200-Calorie Myth".

way more about intake goals and food ideas in later chapters. For now, let's discuss that other thing that goes hand in hand with weight loss: sweat loss.

EXERCISE (EVEN THOUGH IT KINDA SUCKS)

I hate exercise. Well, that's not 100% true anymore. I hated exercise all my life until I recently realized it's my friend. I still don't ever *crave* exercise, but I have actually come to be able to look forward to it. Exercise makes me skinny, it makes me healthy, and it makes me feel good. Sure, it's hard at times, but it's so much easier than life as a fatso was.

When I started losing weight, I chose to exercise only about twice a week, usually two short runs. Since I didn't like exercise, this was more than enough for me. But things changed; when I recognized how beneficial exercise is, and when I saw the results on the scale after almost every time I worked out, exercise became much more desirable. I eventually came to exercise about three or four times a week. I would usually swim twice (for about 40 minutes) and run twice (one short run, about 15 – 20 minutes, and one longer run, 30 – 60 minutes). Sometimes I would substitute a session on an elliptical machine for one of my runs or swims. Exercise can get boring, so mixing it up helps a lot.

Running has always been the most effective weight loss exercise for me, but I've never been good at it, nor did I ever enjoy it. Running is just plain hard—but *gosh* does it ever work! It burns mega calories and it keeps you burning them: you not only burn calories during your run, you have an "afterburn" effect where your body burns fat for hours later. Yeah, it's hard, but it rocks. And it gets easier the more you do it. I no longer feel like I'm going to die when I run—but I sure did at first.

I also started swimming. Swimming actually burns as many calories as running does, but it is easier on your body. The main reason I enjoy swimming is because there's a hot tub to dip in afterward as a reward. It feels like dessert for the body. Swimming also does something running doesn't: it tones muscles all over your body. After swimming, my posture is better. I also feel little compact (and sexy) muscles in my back, shoulders, and arms. Not bulging muscles, just nice little muscles. It really is a serious workout. And just so you know, I am a total crap swimmer. Someday, I will get good at it and quit looking like a dork. In the meantime, I am just happy to be getting healthier. Besides, I'd rather be dorky and skinny than cool and fat.

But all this is just me. The most important thing is that you find the exercise that works for you and, more importantly, that you *like*.

ATTITUDE (THE DIFFERENCE BETWEEN BEING SKINNY AND WISHING YOU WERE)

- *Diets suck. I am not on a diet. Rather, I have completely changed how I think about food.*
- *Food is a tool. It's something your body needs. Fine then: fuel your body. Just don't use food for entertainment or comfort.*
- *Eat what you need, not what you want.*
- *Treat food like you would a prescription drug: if you get in the habit of using more than you need, you're in trouble.*
- *Food can be like an abusive boyfriend: it swears it wants only to make you happy, but in reality it just drags you down.*

The above are just some of the many thoughts I've come up with as I've readjusted to life as a skinny person. I don't know how many will apply to you, but I suspect all of them will.

A weight-loss mindset (or a weight-maintenance mindset, which is the same thing with differing goals—more on that toward the end of the book) is something you're going to have to keep up for the rest of your life if you're going to be successful. That means two things:

1. You cannot think of it as "*A Diet*" that you're going to abandon once you hit a goal. It is going to have to be "*Your Diet.*" That is, not a temporary change in eating, but a lifelong system of maintaining your weight, something you live with and stick with.
2. *Have patience.* Losing weight takes time when done properly. Besides, what's the rush? You're not going to relinquish your new, healthy way of life once you reach your goal, so don't put yourself through misery

on the way there. Make solid changes that you can manage, not drastic changes which will burn you out.

Let me say this again. You need to get the following into your head: THERE IS NO QUICK, EASY FIX. You must choose skinny, it doesn't just happen. AND THERE CAN BE NO GOING BACK. If you think you're going to eat right "for a while" until you reach your goal, and then go back to your old ways, YOU WILL FAIL.

Once more, because you MUST grasp this:

> This is the secret to your success, and that which will put the mockers in their place. When you wrap your head around the idea that this is something you're going to do for life, that getting thin is not like buying a new outfit or signing up for a class, it's not a pill you take until the bottle is empty, it's not a surgery you go in for, but it's a change not just in what you do but in *who you are* … once you know that, my friend, there's no going back. You will be skinny forever.

I invite you—no, I *urge* you—to take a good hard look at yourself. Do you really *want* to be skinny or do you just *wish* you were skinny? I wished I was skinny all my life and it never got me anywhere, unless you count "depressed and loathing myself daily" as somewhere. *If you want it, you will make it happen.* If you're not making it happen … are you sure you want it?

FAILURE: HOW TO DEAL WITH IT & GET BACK ON TRACK

You're human. That means you're going to screw up. I don't know how to help you get past that, but I can share how I have gotten past my own mistakes. Maybe something will make sense.

In the past, when I would screw up (meaning: overeat, fail to exercise, see a higher number on the scale, or most often all of the above), I would just implode into a black hole of self-loathing. Gosh, but have I ever hated myself over and over and over! Now, thanks to the wonderful girls online, I realize that it's not that I'm a BIG F**KING LOSER (sorry to be so dramatic, but that truly is how I have felt time after time), it's just that this stuff is hard, really HARD, and we're all going to stumble now and then. Even the most successful people do.

The truly important question after you screw up is, "*Now what?*" You can go on a big destructive tantrum and beat yourself up, or you can just face the reality that the damage is already done and you're not going to be able to go back in time to undo it. Once you confess that you can't change the past, you can move on and instead change your future.

Ask yourself this question: "*What can I do to reverse the effects of my mistake?*" I guarantee the answer will be, every time, "Just keep on running this race."

Screwed up? *Keep on running this race.*

Making progress but it's taking a million times too long? *Keep on running this race.*

Been trying for days and have seen no results and feel like eating a whole tub of ice cream since nothing seems to make a difference no matter how hard you try? *Keep on running this race.*

Wound up eating the ice cream, purged it all into the toilet, and now hate yourself more than ever? *Keep on running this race.*

Life crumbling around you? *Keep on running this race.*

Because, really, *what will happen if you stop? It won't be success.* The only direction you can successfully coast … is downhill.

Time won't stand still. One year from now, no matter what happens, it will still be a year from now. You can do nothing about that. All you can do is change where you wind up when Today's next anniversary comes around. The only thing that can change where you wind up *then* … is the choice you make *now*. And tomorrow. And the next day. And the day after. It's simple. It's not easy, but it's simple.

2 | Beginnings: Peak of Summer, Peak of Weight

It all began a few days after I discovered thinspo. I realized it was my turn to change. I also feared I wouldn't last more than a matter of hours.

Tuesday, Jul 27

8:40 am – This might actually work!

Hunger is a GOOD thing, not a bad thing! Why has it taken me so long to realize this? – me, today.

Oh my *gosh*, have the past couple of days ever been astounding! I've actually been able to say NO to food, like I've discovered some kind of newfound power! Wow.

Take Sunday, for instance. I went to the beach for a picnic with friends. I had chip duty, and brought large bags of potato and tortilla chips. I didn't eat a single one. Instead, I had a single piece of flatbread topped with some of my friend's homemade guacamole. Then I just sat back in my beach chair, enjoyed the sun, sipped my water, and watched everyone eat. And eat. And eat. They urged me to eat more, to try the potato salad, to have a soda, but I remained unmoved. Of course, I *wanted* to eat. But I wanted skinny more.

Two days later, I'm already down a pound and a half! I've already forgotten what some of the other foods at the picnic were, and I never died of hunger.

This is awesome!!!

Saturday, Jul 31

11:10 am – Saturday breakfast survived!

I got together with friends for our usual Saturday tradition, the $3.99 breakfast special. The horrible thing is, it is SO delicious … crave crave crave!

Today was my first Saturday since I began eating well, and I worried I would succumb to my LUST for this awesome breakfast. But I didn't! I actually did okay!

Usual breakfast:

- 2 fried eggs
- 4 pieces of toast with 2 pats of butter and 2 packets of jam
- an entire sausage patty
- fried potatoes with TONS of ketchup
- 3 coffees with 2 creams each

All told, well over 1000 calories—in one meal! Eek!

Today's breakfast:

- 2 poached eggs (cooked in water, not fat)
- 3/4 of an English muffin … with NO butter and only one packet of marmalade
- 1/2 my sausage patty (I gave away the rest saying, "Here, this is really good, try it!")
- a small cup of FRUIT instead of potatoes (well, truth be told, I had two bites of my friend's potatoes)
- and no cream in my coffee! (that was a tough one, but it spared me 150 calories!)

For a total of about 400 calories! It was still more calories than I would've preferred, but small enough that I can walk it off no problem this afternoon, and not so small that anyone would accuse me of not eating.

Happy!!!

Sunday, Aug 1

9:55 am – One full week since starting

Hunger rocks! I've been doing this for only a week now, but *instead of craving food all the time, I've kinda been craving hunger.* I can't believe I am saying this!

Hunger is cool. Hunger means I'm losing weight. Hunger means I didn't blow it again. Hunger means I *can* have self-control! Right now, hunger is my friend.

Oh, another new thing, so cool, especially right now in the middle of Summer: when I drink from a bottle of cold water, I feel it go ALL the way down and coat my empty stomach with coolness. *So refreshing!* I never used to notice this before because there was always a pile of food sitting in my stomach.

Summary: after one full week of smart eating:

- Weight lost: *four, yes FOUR, pounds!*
- Who noticed: *meeeee!*
- I am feeling: *GREAT and full of hope!* I have a long way to go, but I know this will work if I keep at it.

3:40 pm – Beach notes

Went to the beach. It was really interesting! I now see the beach through totally different eyes. I realize beach bodies are not always so inspiring after all. I saw only one girl who looked amazing, and many who looked decent, but most were actually kinda chubby. Stupid America and our culture of excess!

I have a long way to go before you could call me skinny, but still ... I found myself thinking, "*Why are you girls heavy? You don't have to be! Just quit eating so much!*" This is *such* a total change! For so long *I* have been the one who couldn't stop eating. Yet lately it has been EASY and almost FUN to avoid eating. I feel like I've been given a beautiful gift.

I know it's too soon for me to proclaim success, but I am so HOPEFUL that I will be able to keep this mindset for a long time. Like, forever, if I can.

11:25 pm – Grrr, social eating!

At a barbecue gathering tonight, I ate the least amount of anyone there, but I still ate more than I told myself I was going to. We were having this amazing roasted meat, SO delicious, like a Top Ten Lifetime Experience. I went to the kitchen to get a glass of water, and the meat was just lying there, begging to be eaten. I gave in and grabbed some. Oops.

That alone wasn't so totally bad, but on top of that my friends got me a bottle of a special soft drink they know I like. I tried to share most of it with others, but it, too, added something like 150 calories to an already too-big meal. Crap. We'll see what the damage was tomorrow when I step on the scale.

This is my first setback in a week, and it's a small one, but it certainly took the wind out of my sails. I don't want to slip up anymore. If I permit myself to overindulge, it will become easier and easier to do it again.

Monday, Aug 2

9:30 am – To breakfast or not to breakfast?

Sigh … gained over a pound today. It's more like TWO pounds, because I've been losing a pound a day the last few days. I know nobody really gains TWO pounds of fat in one day, so I'm blaming it on the REALLY HIGH SALT INTAKE I had yesterday (I ate over a cup of salty homemade salsa, thinking it was a good way to get vegetables).

I'm sad, but at least I have a reason to think that everything is okay. If I avoid salt completely for a day or two, I think my body will rid itself of the bloatage.

But today I have another problem: I've been up for an hour and a half and I still don't feel like I NEED breakfast. I think I can last another hour or two before I have to eat. But in the back of my mind, I keep thinking of all the times I've heard people say, *"You mustn't skip breakfast!"* and I think, *"Okay then, here goes …"* Except then I get scared that I'll get in the habit of giving in too soon. I *want* to be hungry—but not if skipping breakfast really does screw a person up.

What do I do?

Sigh.

In other news: I saw this gorgeous thinspo pic this morning: This girl was lying on her back on her bed, sheets all ruffly and gorgeous, her perfectly flat tummy and pokey hipbones bathed in the morning light. It reminded me of when I was at a lower weight. Not that I looked nearly so good, but on days when I felt skinny I would jump out of bed and be so full of energy. The sun shone warmer those days, colors were brighter, flowers more fragrant … I must return to—and surpass—that low weight!

Tuesday, Aug 3

9:10 am – Starvation mode can stuff it

Dunno if I've entered "starvation mode" (can you do that after only a week?) but even after eating well yesterday, I lost only one pound from the one and a half I gained the day before. I had hoped it was all water retention. Maybe it is. Whatever.

I don't care if I AM in starvation mode. It can slow me down, but it can't get around the pure friggin' FACT that if I consume fewer calories than I burn, I win. So kiss my soon-to-be-skinny ass, starvation mode!

2:35 pm – Small victory at the mall

I was walking past the pretzel shop, and a guy was standing in the walkway, giving out samples of a soft, gooey, cheesy pretzel thing. The two people walking in front of me declined a sample, so I smiled at him and said, "You poor thing, you can't even give them away!" He smiled back and started to hand me a sample, but I apologized and said that I, too, was going to be one of the ones refusing his sample today. He seemed happy that someone cared, though.

I continued walking on, and it took me like a full half minute before I realized, *"OMG WHAT DID I JUST DO??? It's two in the afternoon, and I've had barely any food all day—and I still said No!!!"*

I was just elated! I was actually feeling legitimately hungry at the time, and the tiny sample would hardly have derailed my eating for the day, but I just wasn't ready to eat. I didn't *have* to eat—so I didn't.

Two weeks ago, I wouldn't even believe this is a true story. I'd pinch myself—but if this is a dream, I don't want to wake up.

4:00 pm – Worldview changing already?

~~Most of my life~~ All of my life I have looked at the really slender, gorgeous people and thought deep down inside, *"You suck!"* because I knew I would never be slender like that. I know it's shallow, and it's wrong, but it's also human to resent those who have what you don't. Even worse is when others have what you *cannot*.

Today at the mall, the beautiful people were out in full force. There was tons of real life thinspo: supercute skinny girls, elegantly bony European tourists, fitness-fanatic moms with better bodies than most American teens', and one especially cute, fit couple who were both total thinspiration and looked amazing together.

The crazy thing was, today, instead of resenting all these beautiful people, I *admired* them. More than that, when I really think about it, I somehow *identified* with them. It was, and is, surreal. Obviously, I'm not one of them … *but I will be.*

This is one of the profound ways thinspo is changing me:

- I go online; I desire skinny.
- I read people's posts; I think skinny.
- I gaze at thinspo; I *feel* skinny.

Next thing, I look in the mirror to see a fatso staring back, and I think, *"That's Not Me."*

Not for long, anyway.

Wednesday, Aug 4

4:40 pm – Relief

The weirdest thought came to me this afternoon. I was kinda forced to eat more than I wanted to eat at lunchtime, and I was upset that I had unnecessary food sitting in my stomach, and I was just grumpy and frowning. Well, less than three hours later, I noticed that I was starting to feel hungry again, and I was like, *Yay!* Yay, it wasn't actually such a huge lunch that it left me stuffed all afternoon! Yay, my body is going to have to feed on my excess fat instead! Yay, my whole mentality is changing! Waves of RELIEF washed over me and put a spring back into my step.

I then thought more about how RELIEF has accompanied me lately:

- RELIEF from the guilt of knowing I am fat—and that it's all my fault;
- RELIEF from the horror of growing fatter and feeling unable to stop it;
- RELIEF that my jeans, which felt like they were going to split open every time I got into my car, are fitting comfortably again;
- RELIEF that I am no longer alone: I now have all the wonderful people online.

For the first time, instead of using *food* to relieve the pain of my *hunger*, I'm using *hunger* to relieve the pain in my *heart*. And it is incomparably more fulfilling.

6:35 pm – Amazing advice!

Something else amazing happened today. I got the *best* piece of weight loss advice—from the *fittest* person I've ever met. I was sitting on a bench at the park, and this gorgeous man sat down at a bench across from me. I pretended to keep reading my book, but really, I just had to stare. He was wearing a t-shirt and shorts, and I could tell his body was perfectly sculpted. Not bulging grotesquely, just amazingly chiseled. He was also *very* handsome. I immediately thought to myself, *"There's no way this man is not a professional fitness model."*

At the time, I was snacking on a 100-calorie pack of crackers. Amusingly, he pulled out a couple of 100-calorie packs of almonds and also started snacking. I so badly wanted to ask him, "Is that how you stay so skinny? By eating tiny snacks?" but I refrained, too shy to start such an awkward conversation.

Before long, another person sat down and struck up a conversation with the man. It turns out he's a celebrity personal trainer whose photo has actually appeared in several magazines. So not quite a fitness model, but close enough! I joined in the conversation after the subject got onto weight loss, sharing that I had recently begun losing weight by eating less. He replied with something I will never forget:

"As a personal trainer, I shouldn't be telling you this, but … the Number One Most Important Thing to losing weight is DIET, not exercise."

Yeah baby yeah! That's what I'm talking about (*little dance done secretly inside*)!

I mentioned that I had noticed him snacking, and I asked if that was what he typically did. He said yes, he tries to eat a little bit every two or three hours. I asked how big of a dinner he usually eats, and he said only about 500 calories. That's tiny! And this was coming from a quite muscular GUY!

This was such a gift! Right when I'm trying to lose weight simply by eating less, I meet a professional fit dude who tells me I'm doing it the right way! *Thank you!* What a cool and happy moment.

Thursday, Aug 5

9:05 am – Umm . . .

Dear body: WTH?!? I ate super well yesterday, and I lost only 1/10 of a pound. That's like 1.5 ounces. I just don't get it. Too much salt again?

In the past, this kind of thing would have made me just give up and binge. This time, it's friggin' WAR, you damned stubborn fat!

3:10 pm – Thinspo saves me again

Online, cruising through thinspo pictures, seeking inspiration, checking on my peeps. Getting hungry. Try to ignore, but the hunger persists. "*I need food; I must get food,*" thinks I. Get up, walk toward kitchen, see my reflection in the mirror. Reflection looks nothing like thinspo.

FFFFFFFFFFFFFFFF NO, I DON'T NEED MORE FOOD!!!

Hunger gone!

7:40 pm – Beach notes

Went for a walk to the beach, just to be alone. There I was, sitting on the sand, and I was suddenly hit by the absurdity of the fact that I live *minutes* from the beach, but my stomach hasn't seen a ray of sun in years. Because I'm ashamed to wear a bikini in public. How pathetic is that?

Fat people are prisoners to their own bodies. I must break out of jail.

Saturday, Aug 7

7:20 pm – Random skinny thought

There's no such thing as elegant and fat. Isn't that interesting? Almost every word that describes a beautiful, elegant woman means, obviously or not, *thin*. What comes to mind with the description "elegant" hands? Elegant legs? Elegant neck? Elegant collarbones?

It works for other things, too. An "elegant" wine glass has a slender stem and thin construction; otherwise it would be "robust". Elegant shoes, elegant necklace, an elegant dress ... these are all dainty things. Ever picture an elegant dress on a chubby lady? Exactly.

Sunday, Aug 8

9:30 am – Two full weeks

Yay, I finally had a happy meeting with my scale this morning—I lost almost a pound! Because this week started with a spike in weight, the remaining five days got me down to only a little lower than I started. Still, I lost 2.5 pounds. Not bad! That's a total of 6.5 pounds in two weeks! It's a small number, but it's well over a tenth of the amount I want to lose! If I can keep up my weight loss at anywhere near this rate, this will forever be known as the last year I was fat!

- *Weight lost*: 2.5 lbs
- *Total lost*: 6.5 lbs
- *Who noticed*: A guy I see every week at church said, "You've gotten a lot of sun! I didn't even recognize you!" While it's true that I got some sun this week, I think what it really was is that he noticed something different about me and either didn't want to mention my weight or couldn't put his finger on it. Either way, I'll take it as a compliment!
- *I'm feeling*: more hopeful than ever! I ate less this week than my first week but also managed to feel less hungry than I felt the first week. I am learning to love living skinny!

I made it through those scary first couple of weeks, even though I had NO idea what I was doing—perhaps it was BECAUSE I had no idea what I was doing. I was ecstatic about losing weight, yet, unknown to me, changes much more profound than this were just beyond the horizon.

Q&A | Questionable Methods

Short term discomfort and lasting joy or short term pleasure and lasting shame? The choice is yours.

I realize my methods might raise certain eyebrows. I also realize they might not be ideal for everybody. All I know is that I was formerly trapped in a self-loathing, destructive lifestyle of being unable to say No to food. One day, I found strength, and I found my path to freedom. Admittedly, it's an unorthodox path, but I'm just so happy about it that I simply must share it. If you come across something that sounds off, please, just keep reading. I promise, it gets much better

Your ideas about food are a bit warped.

They sure are! The reason I am so ready to admit this is because I spent my entire life trying to make "gradual" changes and to follow the suggestions that "they" made—and it got me nowhere. This time, my entire experience, which I gladly share with you, for better or for worse, is merely *my experience*. I went into this with absolutely NO plan whatsoever (certainly not intending to write a book), only a desire to cut my intake drastically. When what followed right away was serious weight loss, I started learning all sorts of things about myself, about food, about my body. Even my increase in exercise was unplanned. All I'm trying to do here is share the process as it happened, in the hope that someone else can benefit.

Your methods don't seem healthful[6] or positive.

Eating less and exercising more are both things your doctor would recommend if you wanted to lose weight, so I'm leaning on the side of thinking that they actually are healthful and positive. If someone takes this advice too far and goes crazy with it, it's similar to someone not taking any diet advice at all and slowly killing themselves with obesity. The truths behind healthy lifestyles remain the same, regardless of which extreme a person is inclined to embrace.

Didn't you experience adverse effects, eating so little food?

Interestingly, no. My body got used to having so few calories every day that it just resorted to burning fat when it needed extra energy. However, this is likely because I ate *good foods*, mostly vegetables and meat, plus multivitamins, and thus nourished my body.

Where eating too little causes problems is when people eat too many crappy foods, especially carb-dense processed "foods". You see, when your body burns fat, the fat supplies *energy*, but not nutrients. And you need plenty of good *nutrients* in your diet (protein, minerals, vitamins, etc—even fat) for your body and brain to function properly.

When choosing how much to eat, it's important to carefully choose *what* to eat, and be cautious to avoid the "less is more" mentality that sometimes trips up people losing weight. Eating less is only one part of the equation. You still need to take care of yourself.

Is skinny even a valid goal?

Sorry, but it's time for bluntness. Fat people are unhealthy. Fat people more often experience depressive disorders. Fat people are more often passed over for promotions. Others are less attracted to fat people. Others respect fat people less. Fat people miss out on too much of life.

But skinny is magnificent. Skinny is the natural result of be-

---

[6] I use the word "healthful" rather than "healthy" to describe things that are good for you, such as habits or foods. Healthful means "tending toward healthiness in those who partake." Healthy means "alive and well," which is NOT true for most of what we eat.

ing an athlete. Skinny is what little girls are when they're at their cutest.[7] Skinny is what glamorous ladies in evening gowns are. Skinny turns heads. Skinny makes almost everything easier. Skinny … well, the list goes on—and I need not.

None of the above has anything to do with one's worth as a person, nor with any other value judgment. Thus, I believe that wanting to get to a healthy weight, even a weight at the skinnier end of the spectrum, is a reasonable and worthwhile goal for someone who isn't already there.

Being fat or skinny is unimportant. It's what's inside that counts.

True, except when it comes to how others relate to you. I wish people would judge us by our personalities, and not by our looks. But that's not how it works, at least not at first. People will write you off or embrace you, instinctively, by your looks. And if they don't like how you look, they're less inclined to take the time to get to know your personality.

1. Is this wrong? Yes.
2. Can it be changed? No.
3. What can you do about it? Nothing beyond making it easier for others to want to get to know who you are on the inside—by taking care of how you look on the outside.
4. Don't think you should have to? See #2.

Why thinspo?

I like to use the expression, "thin gives life". I don't lightly consider my choice of words. I think it's actually a heavy statement. I choose it to celebrate my newfound power over fat, a vicious foe I have battled since before I can remember. Essential to this battle, for some, is thinspo.

Does not almost everybody agree that we should have goals? Yet how can you pursue a goal when you don't know what the goal looks like? Pictures of gorgeous slender people remind us of how lovely our bodies can be if we are mindful to take care of them. Thinspo touches us with its beauty and re-

---

[7] By this, I mean something along the lines of a young girl with flowers in her hair. She is always the portrait of sweetness. Make her overweight, however, and suddenly painters put down their brushes.

minds us of how gratifying it can be to reach our goals. Some people—and I envy these people—can just decide one day to get into shape, and then get out there and do it. Other of us, however, don't have that kind of power. We need more than to be told, "Get off your ass!" We need instead to be reminded how awesome it would be to *have* an ass! To entice us to keep on working at getting healthy, we need constant reminders of what we can achieve. We need support. We need thinspo.

When you're enveloped by darkness, totally trapped and lost, what do you need? *You need a light at the end of the tunnel.* For some of us, when we are in darkness, feeling trapped in our uncooperative bodies, discouraged and wanting only to give up and eat ourselves into oblivion, *thinspo is our light.*

But isn't thinspo dangerous? Doesn't it trigger those with ED tendencies to embrace a disorder?

The dark side of thinspo shows up when girls use thinspo not as motivation but as measurement, when they won't be happy until they look exactly like the pictures. The problem for such girls is, once they get to a healthy weight, they will seek pictures of even skinnier girls, perhaps unhealthily-skinny girls, convincing themselves that they're, in comparison, "fat". For such girls, it's not the pictures that are the problem.

Thinspo is like medicine: although it causes side effects in some people, within limits it can be quite beneficial. Many people can find motivation without gazing at thinspo. They have been given a gift. They don't need thinspo as a crutch. Some of us do.

4 | Late Summer: Getting Smarter, Getting Skinnier

To my delight and surprise, after weeks of fighting the hunger and the cravings, I found myself neither discouraged nor beaten down but emboldened and encouraged. The lessons in skinny kept rolling in, renewing my mind as they transformed my body.

Monday, Aug 9

8:05 am – Random but empowering thinking

I can look at thinspo all day. I really do love it. But here's a thought: if I lose enough weight, I won't need to go online to find thinspiration anymore—I can just look in the mirror!

Yesterday, I didn't eat 100% awesome (small amounts, yes, great foods, no), nor did I exercise. But I still lost a tiny fraction of a pound. Whew, that was a close one! You really have to keep on top of this weight loss stuff.

Today, after noticing that my hunger is barely ever a problem anymore, I had this weird but inspiring thought: "*Addicts going off drugs have withdrawal problems, but they can eventually become free. YOU are addicted to FOOD. When you quit `using' food, you, too, go through withdrawal—but you, too, can be free.*"

Soon, I will be free!

Tuesday, Aug 10

7:25 am – Super sweet day!

Gosh, I just love hunger. It makes me euphoric! It means I am—for once—in CONTROL of the direction my body is headed! It means the sun is finally shining after an age of cloudy weather.

Like today: I hit a small milestone. I made it into the (ugh) 150s! I am now 159.9! Sheesh, that's still huge, but it is such a relief to have my weight starting with a new, lower, number. It feels like a great victory.

Fat, you can try, but you can't win! I am too determined to DESTROY you.

7:05 pm – Positive

I was asked why I'm so positive about weight loss instead of being all down on myself like many others are.

I thought about it. I realized I'm positive because I am just so OVER hating myself. I did that all my life, and I refuse to go back. I've had enough. I'm ready to release the real me from these self-imposed chains. Even though I still need to lose weight, I don't feel like I'm a fat person anymore. I'm focusing on the pounds I've lost, not on the pounds I want to lose.

It's the same thing with food. I'm over it. I've had years of enjoying almost as much food as I wanted. *That's how I got to be in this mess!* That food didn't give me lasting satisfaction, it gave me deep pain.

I am on my way to enjoying a healthy weight and all the perks that come with it. All it's costing me is a moment here and a moment there of saying No to a what is really no more than a moment of pleasure. *That* is a rockin' deal! *That* is something to get excited about. *That* … is why I am positive.

Wednesday, Aug 11

1:15 pm – Feeling skinny

I've been checking out my reflection, and I've been happy with what I see! As much as I have hated my body ~~most~~ all my life, I can see someone attractive underneath, waiting to shed this disguise. I'm so excited! In fact, I'm going to go get some exercise (did that just really come from *me?*) right now!

Thursday, Aug 12

11:10 am – Thin things

People are friendlier when you're thin. When you're overweight, you walk into a room or make introductions, and people are just like, Hi, whatever. If you're *really* fat, people can hardly contain their contempt.

But when you're slender and attractive, people light up when you enter a room. When you make their acquaintance, they actually look you in the eye and take more of an interest in you. Members of the opposite sex smile at you for no reason—even hot ones!

I noticed this the last time I lost weight. And I've been noticing it again these past few days. People are already treating me better. This increases my confidence ... which makes me friendlier ... which makes people friendlier with me ... which increases my confidence.

I love where this is going! The rewards of getting healthy go far beyond a more pleasant clothes buying experience.

3:35 pm – Eating problem spotted

I've been out of the house every day for a couple of weeks. Hunger comes and goes, but it's never really been a problem. Today, however, is different. I've been sitting at home on the computer and phone all day. *Hunger a problem! Too close to refrigerator! Danger! Danger! Run away!*

I'm going running. Hopefully all I need is some fresh air and some sunshine.

Moral of story: *butts grow when planted.*

5:40 pm – Moments later

Just got back from my run ... OMG it was awesome! It was the first time I've run in about two weeks (I hurt my knee) and it was way EASY! My feet could totally feel that there was less weight pounding the pavement and my flab (hate that word) was noticeably less pendulous (is that even a word?) than it was the last time I ran!

GLEEEEEEEEE!!!

Friday, August 13

11:50 am – Cukecrackers

I can't believe I've never thought of this before! What a delicious snack idea! I had some hummus in the refrigerator and I wanted some as a tiny snack, but I didn't want the carbs from dipping crackers into it, nor did I care to simply spoon it into my face.

Enter cukecrackers!

I sliced a cucumber into thin round "chips" the size of crackers, then dipped them in hummus. It was awesome! What do we even need regular crackers for?

Cukecrackers aside, today was a bit of a blow. I've lost only half a pound in four days of good behavior. I've been eating about 800 calories per day and exercising about three out of every four days. I'm trying to stay positive … but this has cast a bit of a shadow over me. What is going on? Should I eat less? Should I eat more? Should I just ride it out because this is just some little speed bump? Am I actually losing fat but replacing it with muscle? Grrr.

In the meantime, I'm just going to keep on doing what I've been doing and pray it works.

3:10 pm – Let's do this

It's time to put legs to my thin desire. By going for a run.

Sunday, Aug 15

9:00 am – Three week summary

As of today, it's been 21 straight days of smart eating. What have I accomplished?

- Lost this week: 1.5 pounds
- Total lost: 8 pounds
- Who noticed: nobody. School resumes soon, so we will see.
- I am feeling: sad, actually. I exercised six days this week with no binges, yet only 1.5 pounds lost? That's better than nothing, but I am still far too heavy to be plateauing! My only hope is that I have lost fat and re-placed it with muscle due to increased exercise.

Meh. Gonna cruise for thinspo.

Monday, Aug 16

11:30 am – Today is a new day

Well, it's morning, and I'm off to eat well and be healthy today. Breakfast was a small portion of oatmeal mixed with a half teaspoon of almond butter, topped off with a splash of milk. Tasted *really* good and needed no butter or sugar.

Lunch will be a pear and some grapes.

Snack, if needed: 100-calorie pack of cheese crackers.

Then I'm going for a 1.5-mile run in the afternoon (well, to be honest, a mix of running and walking).

Dinner will be mahi-mahi lettuce wraps. It's a new recipe, loaded with veggies, and I can't wait!

6:20 pm – Great run

Instead of 1.5 miles, I ran almost 2.5 today! Woot!
Now I'm beat.

6:50 pm – Dinner success

Wow, the lettuce wraps were even better than I thought they would be. I feel good!

Tuesday, Aug 17

1:05 pm – Plateau doldrums

Still on a crazy plateau, no weight lost in several days. I'm convinced I've gained muscle mass (I can feel more muscle in my legs) and that I am still losing fat, especially because I've gone a little bonkers with exercise the past week. Almost all of the exercise has been running and cycling, which should be helping. I'm bummed, but hopeful.

I wish I could convince my body, "*Look, I'm not going to let you starve! You can keep that metabolism up where it used to be. I'll resume eating more once I hit my goal, I promise!*"

8:15 pm – Binge averted

My temporary dental crown, installed today, just popped out

as I was flossing my teeth. Crap! I tried to use store-bought dental cement to put it back in, but now it doesn't fit right. I can't see the dentist tomorrow, and he leaves the following day for a weeklong vacation. What the hell am I going to do? I know it's going to hurt every time I try to chew. *Stress!*

In the past, this kind of thing would've made me binge. To-night, I'm just going to stay hungry and feel sorry for myself instead of trying to sedate myself with food and drink. That's an improvement, right?

Thursday, Aug 19

8:00 am – Unplateau?

Down almost a pound, finally! I hope this means my plat-eau is relenting.

Today is going to be hard. I am at functions for both lunch and dinner, plus dinner will have wine and fancy hors d'oeuvres that are going to be killer delicious and hard to resist.

I can't screw this up, I've been working too hard.

PS: the tooth problem was averted. My dentist allowed me to come in early yesterday, without an appointment. Whew!

Friday, Aug 20

8:20 am – Unproud

Just made it through several long, stressful days of events and meetings. Each day, I ate an awesome breakfast, really sen-sible lunch (although there were super yummy free lunches, I still stuck with salads), and also each day (aw crap, here we go …), I ate a bit of a splurge-tastic dinner. Not exactly binges, but not as controlled as I've been for the past three and a half weeks, either. I know it prevented me from losing more weight.

Lesson learned: *I need to be super vigilant!* With Summer Break ending, my schedule is going to require some new thinking. I can't let myself think *"I'm worn out, I deserve a treat"*—not when "treats" undo my success.

I'm going to set an alarm on my phone to remind me, each day around dinnertime, that I can't splurge anymore. If I avoid alcohol and keep dinners as small as my other meals, I should be okay.

Saturday, Aug 21

10:15 pm – Better

I had a better eating day today.

- Breakfast: cappuccino and string cheese: 200 calories
- Lunch: a morsel of leftover chicken (skinless white meat): 100 calories
- Snack: veggie burger patty: 120 calories
- Dinner: white fish and salad: 225 calories
- Beverages: a couple of unsweetened iced teas with 1% milk added: 50 calories
- Dessert: spoonful of chocolate ice cream with a maraschino cherry: 30 calories
- Total: 725 calories

Gosh, it adds up fast. Still, I was much better behaved than I was the past few days. Every little bit counts.

Sunday, Aug 22

9:00 am – Four weeks down

It's been almost a month that I've been at this and I'm so happy about it! Before I start my day, let's weigh in:

- *Weight lost this week*: one pound—but that includes three days where I was eating more than planned.
- *Total weight lost*: nine pounds.
- *Who has noticed*: nobody said anything specific about my weight loss this week, but I have gotten a few compliments on my looks in general, which is quite nice!
- *I am feeling*: Unhappy with only one pound lost, but *happier* than I would be with *none* lost! If I'd eaten well all week, it would probably have been two pounds. Nevertheless, I am feeling more room in the hips and thighs of my jeans, and my muffin top is definitely receding!

All in all, I am still making progress, my daily weight graph still shows a downward trend, and in total I have lost more than 20% of what I want to lose. Even if it takes another YEAR before I'm happy with my weight, that's nothing compared to the several years that I've been slowly gaining weight and feeling ashamed all the time. Things really aren't that bad.

2:45 pm – Someone noticed!

My friend noticed that I've lost weight! Yes!!!
Doing my little dance

3:15 pm – Dear Salad

In a fit of silly inspiration, I wrote a love letter.
Dear Salad,

I'm sorry for all those times I ignored you when I was into those other lovers, those pathetic burgers and pizzas and other scum. I just want you to know that I am not seeing them anymore. We're through.

Now that I've been spending time with you again, and not any longer in those abusive relationships, I see you in an entirely new light. You are so amazing. You satisfy me in a way they never could. I want more and more of you every day. I want to get to know you better, to immerse myself in your wonderful ways, to adore you, and to show you how much I love you.

When I'm with you, life is beautiful. You and me, we belong together. I promise to always give you the respect you deserve and to love you until the day I die.

I am yours. Love always and forever,
XOXO

7:10 pm – I love not screwing up

Ate awesome today, including tons of fresh vegetables (I luv you, salad!). I am officially DONE eating today—no matter how hungry I get. I will be going to bed happy and waking up probably even happier after jumping on the scale!

11:40 pm – I made it!

I am going to bed good and hungry … with emphasis on the "good". I am so OVER stuffing myself with food. Food can be such a cruel drug!

Monday, Aug 23

6:00 pm – Running on empty

Wow, I went for a run and GREATLY exceeded my usual length that I could run before needing to stop and catch my breath. I went at an easy pace and I just kept on going! Usually, I am ready to die after five minutes, and I feel quite good on days when I can run ten minutes without stopping. Today: fifteen minutes before stopping, baby!

After that, I kept on running (stopping only once to visit a cat) and it was just *so easy!* I am lighter, so the running is *way* easier. In total, I ran for 28 minutes. This is *gigantic* for me!

It's all working! Not only am I looking better, but other things are getting better! Losing weight is so totally worth it.

11:55 pm – Bedtime bliss

Going to bed HUNGRY like I should. I got hungry *really* soon after eating dinner tonight, which is okay, because that means:

1) My metabolism is fired up from my before-dinner run!
2) I'm going to wake up skinnier!

Tuesday, Aug 24

10:15 pm – Who's lost ten pounds?

I'VE lost ten pounds, as of this morning. This is awesome!

Tomorrow marks my one-month milestone of healthy eating. I lost double digits within the space of that month. That makes me SO HAPPY!

I've lost almost a quarter of what I need to lose to reach my Goal. I don't expect to keep losing ten pounds per month, but I do expect to BEAT THE EVIL FAT MONSTER!

Wednesday, Aug 25

11:20 am – Fat is expensive

For every ten pounds a person is overweight, studies show, that person will make $3000 LESS per year than if they were at a healthy weight. We truly *can't afford* to be fat!

It's about far more than monetary rewards, however. I did the following algebra:

Being hungry means I didn't screw up.

+

Not screwing up means I'm getting skinny.

=

Not being a fat screw-up feels amazing.

Thursday, Aug 26

7:30 am – Feeling skinny today

Awoke to a really nice feeling. My tummy felt somewhat firm and flat (ish) when I got out of bed. The scale confirmed that I had lost almost a pound. I was also fairly dehydrated, so I'm only calling it half a pound. Regardless, I am happppyyyyyyyy!

My plateau is definitely OVER. It lasted about a week, but, true to my predictions, I just kept up the same routine of eating well and throwing in a little exercise. Try as it might, my body simply couldn't prevail against the FACT that more calories expended than ingested equals weight loss! It's so true that anything worth having is worth waiting for.

Things are really turning out nicely these days. Soon, I should be able to fit into my old pair of jeans and throw out my fat jeans! I tried on the old jeans last night. I could get them buttoned, but only with a severe muffin top resulting. Another five to eight pounds and I should be good to go.

Later, as I get closer to my low weight from years ago, I have another pair of jeans (they're so old they aren't even fashionable anymore) that is even smaller! I will *really* feel great (and sexy) when I can fit into them again. And then when I hit my Goal Weight, even those jeans should be too big!

It's so much fun to be thinking about this—*and* being convinced it *will actually happen!*

Friday, Aug 27

7:10 am – Odd thinspo

Interesting! I read an article showing that even doctors recommend "Very Low Calorie Diets" for people who need to lose a lot of weight.

"Next to bariatric surgery, nothing is more effective for weight loss than a VLCD, including pills and other diets," says Dr. John Hernried, medical director for a weight-loss clinic in California. But the diet "is not [for] someone who wants to lose 10 pounds."[8]

All the usual "Do not do this without your physician, etcetera" appears in the article. It mentions how a man lost *233 pounds in a year by eating 800 calories a day!* [And here's the best part!] *"For the most part, I wasn't hungry,"* [he] says. *"I was fine with what I was eating."* That's what I'm talking about! If a 450-pound man can do that on 800 calories, anyone should be able to do it.

This is mighty strange thinspo, but it put some needed spring back into my step! I had been starting to wonder if I should be eating more. No way.

Sunday, Aug 29

5:30 pm – Five weeks in

Five weeks of healthy eating today. Progress has been slow but steady. Isn't that amazing? *Steady!* That is a great feeling, and enough to make up for the way I find the "slow" part of "slow and steady" so frustrating.

- *Lost this week*: 2.5 pounds
- *Total lost*: 10.5 pounds
- *Who has noticed*: A couple of friends today asked me to lunch. They noticed how little I ordered (and ate), and mentioned that I was looking "toned" lately! Obviously, I have a way to go before they say "skinny," but I am happy to be considered "toned" for now!
- *I am feeling*: Quite relieved that my plateau is over!

Plans: take advantage of school days: I tend not to each

---

[8] www.cnn.com/2009/HEALTH/12/15/very.low.calorie.diets/index.html

much at school. I'm only tempted to eat when at home or when partying or eating out with others. So, I will make sure school days are REALLY awesome for food control. That way, I won't have to completely abandon meals with friends.

Also, there's a swimming pool at school. I've decided to try going early in the morning—when nobody should be there to see me in my bathing suit—once or twice a week.

I had made huge progress. The problem was, I was also still rather huge myself. I had so much more to learn about weight loss, about being healthy, about how society can mess with your head, and, to my surprise, about how difficult it can become when people around you start noticing your weight loss.

Q&A | How Much Food are we Talking Here?

*Focus not on how hard it will be to get there
but on how great it will be to arrive.*

How much should you eat? There's no foolproof answer which works for everybody, as the right amount will always vary from person to person. I can almost guarantee, however, that it's going to be a lot less than you've been eating.

Sorry, but it's true. I do have one easy method to make the idea more attractive, however. Go look in the mirror. That's how your current diet has been working for you.

The reason it's hard to embrace the idea of eating less is NOT because you *need* as much food as you've been eating. It's simply because you're *used to* eating that much. When you do finally apply your new thin thinking, and when you do it consistently enough to build new habits, eventually it will *replace* your idea of a what a "normal" amount of food is. Eating less will stop seeming like a sacrifice, but like part of your everyday routine, like part of who you are. And soon, it will *become* part of who you are: a self-controlled, confident, beautiful, slender you.

I know it's not an easy answer, but figure out how to apply it, and you're pretty much there.

Describe your diet?

I don't follow a "diet," and I don't really have a "system" that I can describe. I just try to eat healthful foods, and if they are calorie-dense (cheese, 100 calories per ounce, hello!) I make a point of eating very little of them. I also read a lot of nutrition labels and choose items with smaller numbers on the labels. For example, recently I was looking in my freezer at the various dinner options I had. Most had about 400 calories, but one had only 240 calories. Because I'd already eaten a larger lunch, I chose the one with 240 calories. Pretty simple, really.

The key idea is to aim for a low daily number of calories, and to keep track (at least mentally, but preferably in a journal) of your intake throughout the day. When you do, you tend to select more healthful foods, as you get to eat greater amounts of such foods for fewer calories. It seems hard at first, but you get used to it as long as you don't binge in between.

The food nutrition labels refer to a 2000-calorie-per-day diet. You eat less than half of that?

That number is for an *average* person who has *no need to lose weight*. But remember that this "average" person is an active, genderless adult with a job that keeps him/her/it moving and who regularly gets exercise (actually not all that average after all!). But make that "average person" a *woman*, who like many of us sits on her butt much of the time, and she needs far fewer calories.

There are all kinds of resources online that can help you calculate how many calories your body needs. You can add calories to your daily limit if you're taller, more muscled, or more active, or genetically disposed to burn more calories (and you must subtract calories if you fall on the other side of the spectrum for any of the above). If you're into that kind of thing, have at it.

As for me, physical exams, including blood tests, indicate that I'm totally healthy at my (rather low) caloric intake, so I'm just going to keep on doing what I've been doing. It makes me thin, it makes me happy, it makes sense for me.

How do I figure out how many calories to eat each day (and how many I'm consuming)?

Through trial and error. You try a certain number of calories for a while and see how your body reacts. "They" recommend 1200 for "average" women looking to lose weight. But, as we just discussed, various factors go into such recommendations. *Your* ideal amount may differ.

To determine how many calories I'm eating, I read the nutrition information on food packages. For fresh foods that don't come with information, I look up the information online, or I just guesstimate. It's less important to have an exact tally down to the last calorie, and more important to simply be AWARE of how much you're eating.

Should I count calories?

You don't necessarily need to count with a pen and paper, but some people find that helpful. I just keep in the back of my mind a rough idea of what I've eaten throughout the day. Today, for example, I've had a tiny bran muffin and coffee with cream. About 100+ calories. I've got 60-calorie string cheese for a snack later. At lunchtime, I'll be going to a meeting where food will be served. I don't know what it will be, but I will try to keep it to about 250 calories (400 if it's really delicious). Dinner will depend on how much I eat at lunch. So in a way I count, but at the same time I refuse to be overly strict about it.

How did you avoid going into starvation mode?

I really have to wonder how much this "starvation mode" that we hear about really affects people. I mean, sure, my metabolism slowed down when I quit stuffing my face so much, but I never experienced what I would call starvation mode. I experienced a few plateaus of a week or longer, sure, but generally, the weight kept coming off.

I think the most important thing is that I just never gave up nor gave in. I avoided trying to figure out the science behind it. That stuff never helped me in the past. Besides, the "science" seems to change every few years, anyway.

Do you schedule eating times or always wait until you're hungry?

I don't schedule *when* to eat, but I try to plan *what* to eat. It's sort of the same in the end. I tend to get up around 7:00, and eat a tiny breakfast within 30 to 60 minutes of waking. I then pack two or three small items to take with me for the day. I save my first snack for late morning (10:00 or 11:00) even if I'm hungry before then. I eat another snack or tiny lunch around noon or 1:00, then if still hungry later, I eat another tiny snack around 2:30 or 3:00. However, if I can last until 3:00 without eating, I try to skip the late afternoon snack, because by then I'm then close enough to dinnertime that I can probably wait until dinner before eating.

After a day of controlled eating like this, I can enjoy a slightly larger dinner that feels substantial and satisfying, and I've earned it by staying on the edge of hungry all day. All in all, it takes some effort, but it's totally doable.

How big are these meals and snacks you speak of?

An average day of weight loss would look like this:
- Breakfast: 100 – 150 calories
- Mid / late morning snack: 80 – 120
- Slightly late Lunch: 200 – 300
- Afternoon snack (only if needed): 80 – 120
- Dinner: 200 – 400
- emergency snack if needed: 150

Total intake is usually under 1000 calories, and almost never more than 1200. Plus, I get to eat all day long!

Do you eat after six in the evening?

I don't set strict rules for myself, I just try to keep it small whenever I do eat. Making hard-and-fast "rules" for yourself, like "no eating after six," sounds too much like a diet, too much like setting yourself up for failure. When you set up strict rules and then—as you know you're bound to do—subsequently break them, you feel like you've failed. You're tempted to think, "*I already failed today, I might as well fail big,*" and then binge, turning a tiny setback into a major disaster.

As for me, I eat when I need to, including at any time in the evening that I'm raging hungry. But I prefer to hold off for that late-night going-to-bed-hungry feeling of victory.

I've often tried cutting back on my intake, but it never seems to work.

That was me most of my life. For some of us, "cutting back" is just a crummy euphemism for "trying to go a little easier on the food and hoping for the best." That often isn't nearly enough. What you may need, and what I needed, is not just to "cut back" on the food intake, but to cut OFF your intake at a pre-determined limit.

I've been eating like you suggest, but when I met with a personal trainer, he said I need to eat WAY more. What do I do?

There's no ONE right way to achieve health. His way is probably BEST for someone who has the time and willpower to exercise like crazy and who has the self control to never binge, etc. Someone like ... a professional fitness trainer.

I have read advice of his kind for years. But I'm not one of those people who can do it. I needed to just STOP eating so much, as eating triggered more eating for me. His way is the ideal, I suppose, but my way is the only way that worked for ME, a person who lacks the discipline to carefully plan every meal and exercise all the time.

I don't know what will work for YOU. You *will* learn, however, if you remain patient and keep trying. Keep a journal of your progress, including daily weigh-ins and food intake. Watch for patterns and you pay attention to how your body responds to various forms of intake. Then adjust accordingly. Don't let someone else tell you something different from what your body is trying to tell you.

Fruits and vegetables: include when counting calories?

Fruits: because of their sugar content, I make a mental note of them but, because they are nutritious, I try to permit myself to eat them. So, officially, no, I don't really count them. But in the back of my mind I think, "*Easy, now.*"

Veggies: cram them in. I almost don't care that they have calories because they have so much other good stuff. But I refer here to "real" vegetables like tomatoes, cucumbers, onions, broccoli, and bell peppers, not starchy items which aren't really vegetables, like butternut squash or (God forbid) potatoes.

Remember, just because it grows with water and sunlight doesn't mean it's immediately a trouble-free item to include in your diet. Some fruits like bananas are very high in calories, and can really slow your weight loss. And, just so you know, corn is *not* counted as a vegetable, but as a carbohydrate.

I want to diet hardcore for a week. Will I lose more weight by eating tiny meals or by fasting?

Fasting is never the answer. Assuming you don't pass out, you will be very uncomfortable and your body will try to shut itself down in certain ways. Sorry, but only long-term goals are viable.

I plan to eat more than you suggest, like 1000-1200 calories. Is that too much?

Not at all! That's actually the recommended amount for most women trying to lose weight. I'm just impatient, plus I know I really do have a slower metabolism than most people do.

Then why don't you listen to the professionals who recommend 1200 calories a day?

Many things go into that recommendation. I won't once again go into a discussion of what makes an "average" woman, but do remember that the 1200-calorie recommendation is intended for just that—an average woman. Your height, build, level of activity, and genetics all make a gigantic difference (sometimes to the tune of many hundreds of calories) to your body's daily nutritional needs. If you're not clinically "average," your perfect amount of intake will differ.

The 1200-calorie recommendation includes many factors, even a psychological factor. Less than 1200 calories' worth of food, when you're just starting out reducing your intake, can seem like an amazingly small amount (many restaurant meals have more calories than that in a single dish!). It takes real determination to keep your intake that low. The 1200-calorie recommenders have undoubtedly considered that if they recommend amounts smaller than this, many women won't be able to stick with it because they simply don't have the heart to pull it off. The 1200-calorie recommendation is a conservative "slow and steady wins the race" guideline for the masses, not a medically necessary rule.

The problem is, some of us don't reliably lose weight at that level of intake. Instead of "slow and steady," we experience "Oh crap this isn't working," which is just too discouraging. It makes us want to give up. For me, keeping myself challenged by eating less, and quickly seeing the results, encourages me far more. It breeds more success. But it may not work for everybody.

The other and more important factor in the 1200-calorie recommendation is *nutrition*. Assuming you already have some body fat, your body doesn't NEED 1200 calories to survive. That number is merely a byproduct of nutritionists' calculations. What nutritionists do is determine the *nutrients* our bodies need (vitamins, minerals, protein, fat, etcetera)[9] and then figure out, *based on the foods that the "average person on the street" consumes*, how much food we would need to eat to get those nutrients. They arrive at 1200 calories' worth of food. BUT: if you eat *better foods* than the average person on the street does, you can get all your required nutrients by eating *less food*, with *fewer calories*, thereby accelerating your weight loss.

By the way, I am not making this stuff up. Once again, consider the VLCD, where *men* are put on an 800-calorie diet. These are the same men for whom the usually-recommended amount (for weight loss) is actually *1800* calories per day! Do you think doctors would put people on a diet that doesn't give them even *half* the nutrients they need? Not a chance—they'd be sued for malpractice! What the VLCD doctors do is *plan* the patient's meals to make sure they contain only the nutrients needed to maintain healthy bodily function, and they *monitor* the patient to make sure they're not suffering any adverse effects. *These are the same things I recommend you do.*

Eat wisely. Take care of yourself. Just don't fear that you're committing suicide the moment you dip beneath a somewhat arbitrary number of calories you've heard others say you should consume each day.

That sounds fine in theory, but I'm still unconvinced

I tested my theory, and the evidence surprised even me. Take a look at the chapter titled "The 1200-Calorie Myth" near the end of this book.

---

[9] Notice I didn't mention carbohydrates. Carbs are not so much a *nutrient* as they are *fuel* for your body's "tank". There's a difference. However, when you're eating less to lose weight, your body converts your fat into the fuel that it would otherwise get from carbs. In other words, you don't need very many carbs until you get down to your goal weight.

I lost seven pounds in one week by cutting off calories at around 600 per day. Is this too good to be true?

Not at all! Rather, it sounds just like what happened to me. Some of that weight was probably (TMI warning!) food that was just sitting waiting to be processed that you didn't replace now that you're eating less. And the rest is likely fat loss: because your body is used to burning calories at a pace to keep up with your former level of intake, it's been vaporizing that fat.

However, if your story is anything like mine, your body will soon adjust to getting by on less food, and the weight loss will slow down noticeably. After that, it's just a matter of sticking with your plan until you reach your goal.

Also, bear in mind that 600 calories is *really* hard to keep up in the long run, and it might even malnourish you if you're not eating lots of good, wholesome food. Were I you, I'd up my intake a little and be more realistic about it. You will still reap the rewards of your hard work.

6 | September: On My Way Down

I had never before lasted even a few days, let alone a few weeks, without giving up on any changes to my diet. What was happening to me?

Wednesday, Sep 1

9:30 am – Four-day plateau ended happily

I woke up a pound and a half lighter! I must have been retaining water the whole time I was plateauing, but still losing fat. Now I am officially more than a quarter of the way to my goal. So sweet!

Totally unrelated but fascinating is this crazy news article I read this morning. Apparently, even the Army is getting fat! The Army has had to change its Boot Camp fitness routine because today's recruits are too fat to keep up and are failing basic training because of it! A bunch of generals issued a report outlining the Army's problem, called "Too Fat to Fight". This is insane.

Thursday, Sep 2

7:55 am – "Normal"

Someone just told me I look "normal," and I don't need to lose weight.

I HATE that! "Normal" these days is crap!

I don't want to be normal. I want to be awesome.

2:45 pm – Winning

I am starting to feel like a winner! Breakfast at 6:30 and lunch at noon totaled a miniscule 225 calories. It's now almost 3:00 and I'm not even hungry.

I LOVE how much easier this is than it was when I first began!

3:20 pm – "Between Jeans"

I have a problem. Before I started losing weight, my jeans were almost too tight to wear. Now, they're baggy on me and look rather silly. However, to fit into my old, smaller jeans (without indecent amounts of muffin top spilling over), I still need to lose three to five pounds.

Frankly, this is actually a nice problem to have. Soon I will look great in my old jeans—and I can just BURN my fat jeans!

Friday, Sep 3

8:20 am – Happy

Down, down, down, my weight is going down!!!

7:00 pm – *Maddening diet pill experience*

I hate so many things about our culture. I saw some new diet pills that promised to REALLY WORK, unlike all those other diet pills. They cost $60—*for only a month's supply.*

Are you kidding me? If people would just spend $60 *LESS* on crappy food each month, they'd probably lose *more* weight than with those expensive pills!

Losing weight is hard work. There are no shortcuts.

Saturday, Sep 4

8:00 am – *Skinny shopping fantasy*

When I get skinny, I'm going to go into all the clothing stores where for so long I've wanted to shop, but nothing looked good on me because their clothes look good only on skinny European figures. And this time, it will all fit me properly!

9:30 am – *Exercise vs. eating control*

I've been thinking: exercise is cool and all, but if I'm honest with myself, I know it's not something I can do every other day for the rest of my life. Keeping my stupid mouth shut, on the other hand, is something I can manage for the long haul.

I am loving this new way of thinking!

Sunday, Sep 5

9:30 am — "Between Jeans" revisited

I am actually wearing my old jeans! I was planning to lose those few more pounds first, but all my other jeans and shorts were in the wash and I wanted to get out of the house, so I just went for it.

They felt really tight, especially in the thighs and seat, and I felt like people must surely be shaking their heads at the fatty in the too-tight jeans. Instead, to my amazement, I actually seemed to get more friendly smiles than usual!

Later, being jeans, they did that lovely thing that jeans do—they stretched enough that now they actually fit me fairly well! I still need to lose a handful of pounds before I feel truly comfy in them, but who cares! *I'm in my old jeans that haven't fit me for over a year and a half!* What a triumph!

Next in line, sitting tucked in the bottom of my closet, are my even older jeans from when I was at my former low weight from years ago. *It won't be long, my old friends. It won't be long until we are reunited.*

10:00 am — Six week summary

This week has been good. Slow, consistent weight loss every day except today where I gained a pound (but I think it's just water retention, so I'm going to ignore it).

- *Weight lost:* 2.5 pounds
- *Total lost:* 13.5 pounds
- *Who has noticed:* My old jeans sure noticed!
- *I am feeling:* More like a regular—rather than fat—person!

Very encouraging overall. Going to keep doing what I've been doing.

Monday, Sep 6

9:50 am – War on salt

I'm trying a salt-free day today. Because the last two days I ate salty stuff, and *SCREECH!!!*—the sound of my weight loss coming to a halt.

Wednesday, Sep 8

9:00 am – Pool time

Came to school early today and swam. It was a lot better than my first swim a couple of days ago, when I went at lunchtime and the pool was almost full. Instead, this morning there were like three people. Until I reach my goal weight (which comes with my goal body), I want the pool to myself, basically.

I'm just really glad I got exercise, because this stupid four-day plateau is looking like it will be a five-day plateau (I'm attending a party tonight). This after a week and a half of being lighter and lighter every single day. Silly, silly body ... I really can't tell why you behave the way you do sometimes.

Anyway, next on today's list: eat awesome and try to smile at people.

5:55 pm – So far so good

I have been faithful to eat well, as planned. I bought a fruit salad for breakfast and managed to save half of it for later, which then became my lunch. I have only 1.5 hours to wait before tonight's party and I know I will last just fine until then.

The best part is: with such an empty stomach, I will need only one drink, perhaps two at the most, to become thoroughly, uh, "social," haha.

2:25 am (Next day, technically) – Party report

Well well well, as promised, I behaved! I made up for the small amount of food with a few drinks though ... oops! I actually had three. I was going to stop at two, but someone insisted on buying me one, and I caved. I did try to say "no," but five minutes later, he asked again, so I changed my mind. But with so little food intake, I don't feel bad about it.

Another observation, to my surprise: *I was getting hit on*, by more than one source! I was *not* expecting that! There was far more friendliness, hugging, and contact than I have noticed in a long time. I mean, that's not what does it for me; I have loftier goals than being hit on in a bar. But still, I am feeling more attractive and confident.

Happy!

Friday, Sep 10

11:30 am – 33.333

I *FINALLY* made it past my plateau and dropped a pound and a half in a day!

That means I have now lost 14 pounds, which puts me exactly 1/3 of the way to my Goal Weight of 125. If I can keep it up at this rate (which I don't 100% expect I can do, but I will *try!*), I will be at my goal (and a new lowest weight ever) by New Year's!

So exciting!

Saturday, Sep 11

5:40 pm – Mallspo

Spent all afternoon at the mall, like over five hours, going to really expensive stores like Hermès, Prada, theory, Saks, etc. and trying on clothes generally designed for Skinny Europeans. It was great inspiration for two reasons:

1. Much of the most beautiful stuff looked great in the store—but bad on me. This always shocks me into wanting to get skinny!
2. The few things that *did* look good on me, I wanted to buy, right then and there. Some looked so good I could almost justify the price. BUT: I know if I buy anything now, it won't fit me in a few months, because by then I will be skinny!

Kind of a weird day when I think about it. I bounced between feeling great that I am losing weight and feeling sad that I still have so far to go.

All in all, I am super inspired, because I know the day is coming when I can go shopping and have EVERYTHING look great on me.

Sunday, Sep 12

2:20 pm – Random skinny thoughts

I'm wearing my fat jeans around the house today. They are barely hanging on to my hips without falling down. I know I'm still chubby, but today I feel skinny!

5:00 pm – Stupidity

I can be so stupid at times. Like right now. I know having some muscle will help me look toned and great, and it's generally a good thing to have, as more muscle helps burn more fat.

But: muscle makes the number on the scale bigger. So I'm tempted to avoid exercise, to avoid gaining muscle, to achieve a lower number.

So stupid.

5:30 pm – Eye-opening lesson

Just recalled a memory from some time ago, in my fully fat days. I went to lunch with a group of people, including a [gorgeous] girl and her father, who were both just so good-looking (and both over six feet tall, wow) and SKINNY.

While the rest of us all ordered burgers and fries, these two ordered a grilled chicken salad—and SHARED it. I couldn't believe my eyes! I exclaimed with amazement, "So *that's* how you're so slender!" Yep, they said, they control what they put in their mouths.

All along I had assumed that they were just some of those lucky skinny people who get to eat whatever they want! But no, it takes mega self-control.

Just like I have been learning.

5:40 pm – Epiphany?

I can't believe that in our modern, sedentary culture, people still believe that a plate of food—a whole PLATE!—is a normal meal. That is just so wrong.

Monday, Sep 13

10:30 am – Feeling skinny

Last night in bed, lying on my back, I had this awesome sensation: my tummy was lying so flat it felt like it was sort of "going into" my abdomen, like in a concave shape. I reached and felt it with my hand. Turns out my tummy wasn't actually concave, but it *was* quite flat. Well, it was lumpy and flat, if that makes any sense. But at least it's flat when I'm on my back!

Next step: concave when I'm on my back.

And then someday completely flat when I'm standing up(!).

It is *so* much fun to think of stuff like this! There are so many gratifying milestones along the way in addition to the lower numbers on the scale (PS—the number *was* lower today!).

Tuesday, Sep 14

7:15 am – Another plateau vaporized

After that very frustrating weeklong plateau, I'm down two and a half pounds in only five days!

It's so important to just hang in there when times are tough.

4:40 pm – Reflections

I was thinking about the weight I've lost, and I was wondering if I am someday going to gain it all back again. I realized I don't need to fear, for several reasons.

1. This time, I'm not on a "diet".
2. This time, I'm not planning to revert to "normal" eating upon reaching my goal.
3. This time, I have learned to feel good about self-control, not just feel bad about eating.
4. This time, I haven't just changed my routine. I've changed the entire way I think about food.
5. This time, *I'm really going to make it.*

Wednesday, Sep 15

9:05 am – Good times

Yesterday's self-control really paid off! Result: down another half pound!

2:25 pm – What's up, hunger?

It's amazing how I'm rarely hungry anymore. When I began, hunger *assailed* me at every turn. It's been almost two months now, virtually binge-free (only a couple mini-binges, like maybe 1200 calories) and things are different: hunger has largely subsided! I think my body has gotten used to eating small.

Unlike in the beginning, when I would get hungry every couple of hours (or less) and I would have to fight it so bad, my hunger is now mild even after four or five hours, and it doesn't make me feel sick anymore. VERY HAPPY about this!

Minutes later

Just saw myself in the bathroom mirror. Guess who's noticing collarbones and [that pointy front shoulder bone] showing up a little better? Wheeee!

8:45 pm – School: good but bad (but good)

Good: I came to school early today and swam for 45 minutes!

Bad: I have been at school for *fourteen* stupid hours and my brain is so fried I just need to go home and crash … and then get up for an early class tomorrow, sigh.

More good: I have been too busy to notice that I skipped dinner. Now it's too close to bedtime to need to eat!

Thursday, Sep 16

7:05 am – Skinny reflections

I awoke feeling skinny, and I definitely liked my reflection this morning! The scale reflected only a fraction of a pound lost, but maybe I have muscle from yesterday's swimming? Regardless, my tummy is looking way flatter. Hooray!

1:15 pm – Pizza "binge"

I got to binge on pizza with zero bad effects!

Okay, I know this sounds anorexic, but it's not. I forgot my healthful lunch at home today. Thankfully, there was a ton of *really awesome* pizza leftover from a student club meeting, and I was allowed to have as much as I wanted.

My first thought: *"Crap! Pizza! The enemy! Run away! Nooooooooo!"*

Still, I ate a slice, because I needed to eat *something* … and OMG it was some of the most amazing pizza I've ever had. I craved MORE! But I knew I couldn't afford the calories.

Solution? I took two more big slices, but then I just chewed them up and spat them out into the trash instead of swallowing.[10] I got to enjoy a huge pizza lunch, but I didn't binge!

2:30 pm – If this is what skinny feels like, bring it on

Even though I have lost only about a third of what I need to lose, I already feel so awesome. I no longer feel like a pig, I feel only "somewhat chunky" these days. It just gives me butterflies to think, *"If I look this good now, what will it be like when I actually AM skinny?"* It's so exciting, I could burst!

This is surely going to be one of the most rewarding things of my life.

Thursday, Sep 17

11:30 am – Milestone approaching

Less than a pound to lose until I am into the 40s (as in, the 140s)! And then, awesomely enough, I will be exactly 40% of the way to my Goal Weight. Progress!

---

[10] Be warned: this is NOT a valid way to lose weight, and it's often a sign of anorexia. Plus, if you try this without actually eating (unlike how I did eat a slice before spitting out the remaining slices), it screws up your stomach, which thinks it's getting food and starts the digestion process … but has only itself to digest (ew!). When you see any questionable behavior in this book, please just keep in mind that I didn't know what I was doing when I first started out. But, if you finish the book, you *will* know what you're doing, and you'll be without excuse if you engage in such reckless behavior.

On top of that, I'm entering a 5K race! It's a few weeks away, but I just signed up and paid, so it's official. I am excited, because by then I expect to be a fair bit lighter—and the running should be way easier.

I would NOT have chosen to do this 15 pounds ago.

Saturday, Sep 18

7:15 am – New thinking

It's so amazing how my attitude toward hunger has changed:
Old days: *"Hungry! World about to end! Must eat!"*
These days: *"Hungry. It's about time!"*

8:00 am – More new thought

Last night, after polishing off a big salad for dinner, I realized something so cool: now that I'm controlling my intake, I eat better foods, because I can eat MORE of them for the same number of calories! What an unexpected side benefit!

I never used to care about stuff like this. In fact, I would *never* choose salad if I could instead choose a burger and fries. But now, knowing that I can't just eat whenever I feel like it, I'm eating a zillion more vegetables and low-calorie, high-fiber foods—because I can cram way more of them into me without overdoing my caloric intake.

I literally laughed when I realized this. *I'm eating LESS food—but getting MORE of the foods I should be eating.* And it's pretty much an accident!

3:10 pm – Even more thoughts

Ate breakfast six hours ago.
Went for a run two hours ago.
And I'm just now barely starting to get a *little bit* hungry! I LOVE this! I thought that by now I'd be burnt out from good eating, but it just seems to be getting easier!

4:10 pm – Something smells

Why is it that you always see articles on eating disorders where they mention "these poor girls wanting to be thin because of societal pressure"? What nonsense! I don't want to be thin because of societal pressure, I want to be thin because *thin is BEAUTIFUL!* The pressure, if any, is to AVOID trying to be thin. We're taunted at every angle by food advertisements, and those of us who are trying to become thin get *major* grief from others. Grrr!

Sunday, Sep 19

9:20 am – Week Nine Progress Update

It was an amazing week! I experienced no meaningful plateaus, only a couple of tiny bumps! It was so much better than last week—which was so frustrating that I didn't even bother with a weekly progress update.

- *Weight lost*: three pounds! This dropped me into the *forties!*
- *Total Lost*: more than 17 pounds.
- *Who noticed*: I've gotten a few compliments on how I look but no "Wow, you've lost weight!" comments. I will infer, however, from the fact that I was getting hit on the last time I was at a bar, and because the gorgeous skinny people at school no longer ignore me when I talk to them, that people don't really see me as a fatty!
- *I am feeling*: wonderful! I'm 42% of the way to my goal!

6:40 pm – Major changes

I really feel like I have achieved the "impossible". I've actually changed how I think about food, from something I worship to something I allow. Previously, I really didn't believe it could be done.

I still *like* food … but I no longer find myself thinking, "*Yum, what's for dinner?*" What actually comes to mind is, "*I guess I'm going to need dinner.*" This wasn't a conscious attempt to re-shape my thinking; it is just the natural result of week after week of choosing not to yield. It is completely unexpected—and totally welcome.

7:30 pm – The shuffling of the shirts

I just went through my closet and discovered that:
- Four of my tops are now too big to wear!
- Seven older tops which were buried in the "I'm too fat to wear these anymore" pile *now fit me again*, including one really nice item that I wore only once (job interview) before getting too fat to wear it.
- Three old pairs of pants now fit me again. I need to wear them like crazy for the next several weeks—because I know that they, too, will soon be too big to wear!

Monday, Sep 20

6:05 pm – Thinspo does it again

I don't really *need* thinspo anymore, now that I've learned to eat better—but just now it worked for me again! I was getting a big appetite (not so much hunger, just an appetite) when I caught some awesome thinspo, and suddenly I want that body incomparably more than I want food. I love this!

I'm going to keep cruising through thinspo. I am SO ready to go to bed hungry tonight and awake to lightness!

8:40 pm –Daydream inspiration

Just had the *best* daydream after seeing this amazing picture of a girl lying on her back on her bed, prominent hipbones and ribs framing a flat, flat—really, concave—tummy. I floated away, imagining what it would be like to have that body:

> Lying on your back, running your hands over your body … luxuriating in the tightness of your skin over your tummy, marveling at how there's so little give when you press against it … rest your fingertips on your ribs and pause there to breathe in … out … in … out … you ponder your ribs' graceful ebb and flow, perfectly synchronized like young trees swaying in a breeze … your hands meander below to the small of your back—so tiny and arching

so high!—and your heart skips a beat as you feel a little spark of delight, thinking, *that's really hot, isn't it?*, as your fingers brush against the deep contours of your spine … you gently lift your hands to your towering hipbones and take refuge in their sturdiness, awed by the regal strength with which they guard your most delicate parts … you smile as you wonder how you can take so much pleasure from such a tiny area of your perfect body … you softly take in a slow, deep breath and let it out in a long, happy sigh … you know, you really know this time, from your own experience … it was all worth it.

Tuesday, Sep 21

8:00 am – Surprise!

Last night, I didn't go to bed hungry after all—because I wasn't even hungry! So weird! All I had for dinner was some cucumber and hummus, not even very much, and I was fine! Stomach empty, yes, but hungry, no. It's hard to believe how little I now need to be satisfied.

Wednesday, Sep 22

10:30 am – Workout wonders

I actually found a workout that makes me feel *better* instead of making be feel *beat*! I went swimming again this morning and couldn't believe how good it felt! Exercise usually makes me feel gross and tired. Running, cycling, tennis, and *especially* using weights in a gym. But the past couple of times I've gone swimming, I've actually felt really good after!

Today, walking back from the pool, I just found it so easy to stand up straight, to keep my shoulders back, to breathe deeply … even my walking stride somehow felt powerful and athletic. If this keeps up, I know I've definitely found my favorite way to get thin and toned.

By the way, none of this is because I'm any good at swimming. Today, while I was rocking my most furious freestyle stroke, the girl in the lane next to me blasted swiftly past me, doing easily twice my speed … and *she was only kicking!* I felt so lame.

But I didn't care, because *I'm getting skinny.*

1:25 pm – It's working

Wow, I can already feel new muscles from this morning's swimming. This means I am going to be a little bit heavier on the scale, so I'm promising myself that I will not freak out. Such is the only time gaining weight is acceptable.

Sometimes, you have to judge your progress by something other than the number on the scale. Today, for example, I'm pleased to report that my double chin is now more like one and a quarter chins, yay!

3:45 pm – Ponderings on normality

When I was fatter, people told me I looked "normal" or "fine"—but I knew I wasn't, and they did, too. Now, at my current weight, I actually DO feel like my body looks "normal".

However, *I am NOT content to be normal.* I ~~want to be~~ must be *thin.* But still, "normal" is SO much better than "fat" that it feels *wonderful!* These days, I'm merely *uncomfortable and unhappy* with my body instead of *disgusted and ashamed* of my body. That is a real improvement, and one I notice every day.

Even better, I can't help but wonder how I will feel when I actually reach *thin.* That thought has been exciting me so much that it's legitimately been keeping me up. I've barely slept the last two nights because I've been so excited about it. I already feel like I'm living the dream. So far, I'm dreaming in black and white instead of in full color, but it's still a dream I don't want to end.

9:10 pm – Bedtime milestone

Today was the first day in my life that I expended more calories exercising than I consumed in food!

TA DA!!!

Thursday, Sep 23

9:45 am – Not panicking

As promised, I'm not going to freak out that I was only a tiny fraction of a pound lighter today. I know I have extra muscle from the vigorous swimming I've been doing. Frankly, it's really nice swimmer muscle, not bodybuilder muscle, so I quite like it.

But ... it still bums me out. At this stage, my happiest days are still the days when the number on the scale drops by a ton.

I know one of those days is coming soon.

Friday, Sep 24

8:00 am – Frustration

Body, how do I hate thee? Let me count the ways ...

Last week, you gave me total bliss as my weight dropped like a rock every day. This week, I've behaved even better, but my weight hasn't budged.

Bleh.

I'm going for a run. I've got to do something to tell my body to wake the hell up and start shedding fat again.

3:45 pm – Goal prioritizing

Been thinking about my goals. Right now, as silly as this sounds, skinny is what matters most.

After I get skinny, I'll be able to fully give myself to the more important things in life, only no longer as an emotional cripple.

9:45 pm – Finally, someone noticed

My friend from school mentioned today that she has noticed I have "slimmed down a lot." Like, DUH, what took you so long!

I'm just so glad someone finally out-and-out said to me that I have definitely lost weight. That seriously rocks.

Saturday, Sep 25

5:30 pm – Happy

I noticed I have really been HAPPY lately! I even noticed that I am appreciating things I used to take for granted. It's like my entire outlook on life is changing. Not only am I happy that I've finally found how to control my eating, and that I'm getting skinnier / fitter / more attractive, but seemingly everything is better. I am quite high, really (but I've never taken drugs in my life!)

Take yesterday's run, for example: I know I live in a gorgeous area. It really is a gift living here. Yet, for years I have gone for jogs around my neighborhood and not even noticed its beauty. Not coincidentally, for years I've also been really unhappy about my ability to do anything about my weight.

Yesterday, however, I was just so happy to be out running, happy that running has gotten easier, happy that this week THREE different people mentioned that I've lost weight ... all of a sudden, I was just blown away by all the beauty around me. I felt absolutely *dreamy*, it was so blissful. When I got home from my run I actually dashed inside to get my camera, then ran back out to take pictures, because I didn't want to forget the moment.

I couldn't believe I had formerly failed to notice all the beauty because I was under clouds of gloominess all that time. Thank God, those clouds have lifted and the sun now shines warm and bright.

Today has been especially good. I was so happy about being happy that I was inspired to go for another run! I just don't get it. This is so cool! I even figured out a silly way to express what's going on: *"Things look brighter when you're lighter."*

Sunday, Sep 26

8:00 am – Week Ten Summary

Very ironic week. I am slimmer than ever, I got more compliments than ever, I feel better than ever, and I've been super thrilled about my weight loss.

But my weight didn't budge at all.

I am going to have to chalk it up to:

1) gaining muscle and
2) weirdness. Mostly weirdness.

Am I frustrated? Quite. Am I going to say, "Screw it, I'm bingeing!"? Not anymore. That was the old me. The new me isn't giving up no matter how hard this becomes.

2:00 pm – Lovely friend moment

My skinny guy friend (more like a cousin than just a friend) hugged me after not seeing me in over a month. He seemed startled with surprise. He was like, "*Whoa!*" and then patted my back and sides (again, not your ordinary friend) as he commented on how much skinnier I've gotten!

Even a while later he was still going on about it, "Seriously, that hug felt *different!*"

Now THAT is the kind of weight-loss noticing I've been waiting for!

9:10 pm – I came up with another silly phrase

"*Lose weight; find life,*" It's silly—but it's exactly what's been happening to me.

Monday, Sep 27

9:25 am – Inspiration through imagination

I saw this amazing photo where beautiful morning sunlight was streaming into a forest, trees' leaves breaking up the light into thick beams reflected by the early-morning mist. I had another long moment of daydreaming about what life will be like when I'm thin.

> Standing here, all alone, everything still all around you ... take a deep breath of cool, delicious morning air and feel it go all the way to the bottom of your lungs ... you slowly let it all out as your stomach deflates flatter and flatter like it could almost disappear ... you're slender and have perfect posture, your arms hang flatly at your sides ... you tilt back your head to expose your face to the sun ... you

feel the skin stretch tautly across your neck and cheekbones, soaking in the warmth of the gracious sunlight … your breathing and pulse slow until you could almost release your spirit with every exhalation … you feel, overwhelmingly: gratitude, lightness, peace.

9:00 pm – Another compliment!

Another friend noticed I'm skinnier! We were at school, and we started talking about swimming, because he noticed me drying my towel on a chair. I stood up, and his eyes bulged a little and he said that the swimming has "really been working" for me!

I wanted to hug him! It wasn't quite the right moment for it, but I made sure to smile hugely and thank him.

Oh! More good news: in less than a month, I have tripled the distance I'm swimming!

Tuesday, Sep 28

7:40 am – Insane-iest plateau yet

Wow. Day Ten of my weight not budging. I know I've gained muscle, but not ten days of fat loss's worth of muscle!

For virtually every day for over two months, I've consumed below the number of calories consumed by my body's resting metabolism, and this last ten days has been no different. I have even exercised five of those last ten days. Still nothing.

Crap happens, I guess.

I'm going to keep doing what I've been doing. This can't last forever. But skinny *will* last forever … because once I get there, I'm making sure I never have to go through this crap again.

9:30 pm – Things must change

I badly need to plunge through this plateau I'm stuck in. I'm going to try a tweaked version of the "Ten-Day Challenge," which is this thing I've seen floating around online. I think the original is too hard (I'd rather not have to keep it up for ten whole days) and too easy to fail (if you don't do everything perfectly every day, you fail). So I'm making a "Seven-Day Challenge" instead (one week to get sleek).

The idea is, every day for a week you eat super strictly and exercise hard while drinking plenty of water and getting a full night's sleep. Each behavior is assigned points, and you try to reach a certain number of points by the end of the week. I think it might actually work. In fact, I'm already ahead in points!

Wednesday, September 29

11:30 am – Things are going swimmingly

I swam this morning for about forty-five minutes, which is HUGE. I just feel so proud of myself. Soon after, I got hungry, way earlier in the morning than I usually do. This is a good thing, as it probably means my metabolism is absolutely raging right now.

I'm liking this swimming business, which is something I've never before enjoyed. It's a little like flying. I hang out in the deep end, which has me soaring more than a dozen feet above the bottom … it's one of the only exercises that can feel serene at times, a little bit like flying.

Thursday, September 30

9:15 am – The plan seems to be on track for success

The Seven-Day Challenge seems to be working, because after ten days of plateauing, I've finally started losing again! I'll wait 'til tomorrow to confirm that the weight loss is real, but I am VERY encouraged. The floor seems to have fallen out of my plateau!

11:00 am – Technology to the rescue

Amazing! I took a friend's advice and downloaded an exercise app for my new phone. After, I went to the gym and got on the elliptical machine. The exercise app was running, and I was simultaneously streaming awesome workout music from the internet.

Holy, I just about ripped that machine apart! For some reason, I was just *pumped*, and having such a blast! I usually hate exercise machines, but today I felt like I was on top of the world. The exercise app was recording how far I had gone and how many calories I was burning, and this soothing voice would come on over my music and report my progress (*"Nine minutes ... fifty-five calories."*). Had I been outside instead of on a machine, the app would even have used GPS to make a map of where I'd gone. Is there anything about this that is not just SO COOL?

2:55 pm – Achieved another impossible thing!

I never thought I could *EVER* (I can't stress enough how much I mean *EVER*) enjoy exercise, but lately that has changed! How impossible is that?!?

I used to eat much and exercise little. I saw virtually no results from exercise, so I was like, *"Why do this to myself? It feels bad and doesn't help!"* The problem was, my exercise couldn't keep up with my eating.

Now I eat little and exercise ... well, still only a little. But *now*, the exercise is actually *doing* something! It is making me skinnier, happier, healthier ... and, due to those reasons, it's getting *easier*. Add everything up and suddenly I find myself LOOKING FORWARD to getting exercise, and enjoying it, and doing *more* of it, because I *want* to, not just because I *need* to.

I expected my weight loss plan would help me *look* like a new person, but I had no idea it would begin to *make* me a new person!!

BLISSSSSS!!!

After more than two months of serious changes, I was still really just beginning to learn how different my life was to become. I had merely wanted to cease being fat; instead, I discovered a whole new world.

Q&A | Exercise

Not always fun: deciding to exercise. Always fun: seeing the results.

Controlling your eating is the absolute most important factor in reaching a healthy weight. There really is no other way, unless you're a professional athlete who works out for hours each day. Nevertheless, exercise is amazing. It's amazing for your weight loss, for your health, and for your ability to enjoy life to its fullest.

What's the best exercise for losing weight?

Lift your lower jaw until your teeth are gently touching. Hold for as long as you can.

Just kidding. But seriously ... it does kinda help.

I have no idea how to get started. I'd like to exercise, but I'm really, really, unfit.

You get started with just a little at a time, and then it gets easier as you get lighter and fitter. Soon, you'll remove one "really" from your "really, really unfit" description. Later, you remove the next "really". And then the "un". Then, once you're left with just "fit," you'll start putting back the "really".

It really is that simple. It sucks at first. But the new you will be *so* glad you did it.

Three or four days of exercise per week seems like too little. How important are rest days?

I've almost never exercised more than four days in a week, and I've done very well with weight loss. Don't underestimate the value of resting your body ... and don't overestimate your ability to exercise hardcore all the time, especially into the future.

Running is so hard. Are some of us just Born to Walk?

The difficulty of running is one of the things which make it such an amazing exercise. Take heart, however: it DOES become easier, even for those of us who aren't naturals. In fact, it can become fun—no, seriously, I meant that!

If you are truly curious, take a peek at Appendix B. There I explain how to get started (in greater detail than I can fit into this space).

How good of a workout is swimming compared to running?

It's about the same, as far as calories spent.

Pros: It's generally easier on your body than running is. It also tones and exercises more muscles. When it's cold and dark out, it can be far more enjoyable to dip into a warm, lighted pool than to hit the mean streets on foot. It can also be very rhythmic and relaxing.

Cons: To some people, rhythmic and relaxing equals way too boring. It also lacks a way to read a magazine or watch a TV show like you can do when on a treadmill / stationary bike / elliptical machine / stair climber / whatever.

In conclusion, if you enjoy it, do it! Finding a form of exercise you *enjoy* is the single most important thing. If you choose an exercise for its efficiency but you hate it, you're not going to be able to keep it up long-term. And skinny requires long-term.

You started out just eating less, but then you got into exercise. Are you now more fitness-oriented?

I know that many people who lose weight with exercise get really into it after a while, and start to focus on abs, arms, and other muscles. I'm not one of them. I have to confess that I am less interested than ever in doing any of that muscle-toning stuff. I just want a flat stomach and a smallish butt, pretty much, and I know I can have that simply by eating right and getting a mild amount of exercise.

Is it better to work out in the evenings or in the mornings?

Some people say you should work out in the morning, because that revs up your metabolism all day (but doesn't doing it at night rev up your metabolism all night?). Then again, working out in the morning makes you hungry sooner in the day, tempting you to eat more. It's all so silly. Newspapers and magazines like to quote "studies" that say you can lose more fat by Tip X or Tip Y, or by working out at such and such a time, but really, the only way you stay healthy is by establishing good habits until they become part of your lifestyle.

As for me, I prefer daytime exercise, because I just don't like things dark. But sometimes night is the only time working out fits into the schedule. Just do whichever you enjoy more. Don't sweat the small details, just get out there and sweat—at whatever time you can.

But you should try to rev up your metabolism, right?

So many people use these bizarre strategies, trying to somehow "trick" their bodies into shedding weight. The most reliable, long-term way to lose weight is to eat lightly and exercise moderately. Most of us are already exercising too little; do you really want the extra stress of struggling to fit in exercise at times when it feels unnatural? The best time is the time you *most enjoy* exercising, because that means you will actually *do* it.

Besides, do you even know how a "revved up" metabolism compares to a normally-revving metabolism? The studies don't necessarily mean much, because for a study to be able to claim a "result," it only requires a tiny, barely measurable effect in a small group of people. Are you willing to play games and jump through hoops and put all kinds of burdens on yourself just to take the chance that you might experience such a tiny benefit?

Find what works for you, and you will be well on your way to skinny. What will *really* get you revved up is seeing regular results from your own honest work.

My running is getting easier, just like you said! It's time to take things up another notch. Should I be working on going faster or going farther?

Faster and farther are both valid running goals. Your personality probably dictates which should be a greater priority. If you like to charge hard and challenge yourself, speed might be a more rewarding goal. It does feel pretty awesome to look at your stopwatch and see a new record. But distance is cool, too: it's immensely satisfying to learn that you can run for a long time, longer than you ever felt possible before. Also consider this: running faster gives you a slightly more toned and athletic build, whereas running farther gives a more leanness-producing fat-burning workout.

As for me, I like to mix it up: when I'm feeling up for a challenge, I try to go fast. Also, in times when I'm not really in the mood to spend much time exercising, a fast blast can be completed quite quickly. It's also a great way of blowing off steam when I'm feeling stressed or wired. But there are times when I just want to get away from the house and get outside, or when I feel the need to be alone for a time. In such moments, distance running is just the ticket.

One more thing: I found over the months that whichever I tried to work on, speed or stamina, both would improve. As I increased my distance, my speed naturally—nay, *accidentally*—increased. When I spent time going hard to become faster, my lung capacity increased, which made the long runs easier. No matter which you do, it will become easier and more rewarding.

What does it mean if I'm sore the day after a workout?

Soreness comes and goes. It depends on how hard you push yourself. Generally, each time you do harder or more frequent workouts than you're used to, it hurts the next day. This can be a good sign, but if you're sore all the time, you should give your body more rest, or you might injure yourself and become unable to exercise at all.

These days, I'm rarely sore after a workout anymore, which I take as a sign of being in better shape. But if I go too many days between runs, I will be a little sore after the next run, which tells me that I lost a little bit of muscle tone.

In general, I wouldn't worry too much; just keep it *fun* so you can continue doing it well into the future.

I have a home exercise machine, but it's just so boring!

Can you read, listen to, or watch anything at the same time?

Cardio machines kill me, too, unless I have a magazine to read or TV show to watch. Beyond that, it's just a case of either:

1. Experimenting to find what other exercise you enjoy; or
2. Choosing the pain of exercise over the pain of fat.
3. (Technically, you can lose weight without exercising if you eat smartly enough. But exercise has so many other benefits, it'd be a shame to go that route.)

All exercise bores me. I prefer to just dance around, listening to music. Is that okay?

Absolutely! Running is simply what works for *me*. What works for *you*, apparently, is dancing—so *dance*! Remember, the more important factor for weight loss is minding what we EAT. It should be small, it should be healthful, and it should be because you *need* it, not because you just *want* it.

I started running weeks ago but still can't last longer than two minutes. If zombies were chasing me, I wouldn't make it out alive.

If two minutes is all you can do ... do two minutes! Seriously, just do what you can. I bet if you walk for a couple of minutes to catch your breath, you'll be able to resume running for another two minutes. Keep this pattern up for a while, and soon you will have had a long workout and burned a ton of calories. The total duration (including the walking parts) of your workout matters far more than how much you can run before you need to walk. And do take heart: eventually you will get good at it, possibly sooner than you expected—and almost certainly before the zombie invasion.

I'm taking a trip to a snowy destination where there's no exercise equipment. How do I still get some cardio in?

I have an odd but cheap idea. Jumping rope is the perfect remedy. It's good aerobic exercise and is even more portable than running shoes are, plus you can watch a show while doing it.

As mentioned above, dancing around and being silly to loud music works, too.

I'm ready to lose tons of weight by working out like CRAYZAY {slobber, slobber, slobber}!!!

Exercise is awesome in many ways, and obviously I encourage you to get out there and do it. But it can be hard to keep up, especially when family, career, emergencies, and injuries intrude into your life. Someday, guaranteed, you will find yourself having less time or energy than you now have. Also, exercise can get just plain boring at times. Being skinny never gets boring— and the easiest way to get skinny is by eating less and by eating better.

But I don't want to eat less. Shouldn't exercise should be enough?

Unfortunately, for many (most?) people, there come times in life when for whatever reason, you are no longer able to exercise as much as you did before. If you were relying on exercise to keep you slim, you will then start to pack on the pounds. The solution?
Either:
1. Never get bored, burnt out, busy, sick, or injured; or
2. Learn to control your weight by controlling what you eat.

Fat lost through exercise often returns when the exercise ceases, and it's all but guaranteed to return if exercise is the only thing you're doing to lose weight or maintain your weight. Weight lost through discipline and good habits in your diet, however, generally fails to return unless you actively increase your food intake. With the right attitude, that is something you can avoid for the rest of your life.

In summary, exercise is good. Unfortunately, it's just not enough.

Fine. I realize I need to exercise. But I still don't like cardio.

Some people love to do strength training, like weights or natural body weight routines like Pilates or yoga. While that's not exactly a substitute for cardio exercise, it does burn calories. It also gives you more muscle tone, which helps make you look hot while also making your body burn more calories throughout the day.

Muscles, just by being there, require food energy to maintain, even when they're not doing anything. Having more muscle means you burn more calories every day, even on days when you don't exercise (you have to admit, that's a pretty attractive reason to build muscle). Muscle tone also makes you less likely to get injured from twisting, lifting, and other innocent daily activities.

Personally, I must confess that I hate strength training. I did it for quite some time, and, although I did like the look of the toned parts of my body, I just got so *bored.* Sadly, the moment I stopped going to the gym, all of my muscle disappeared, taking with it my spirits. But if this kind of exercise does it for you, then hey, lift on!

Also, don't forget the value of competitive and recreational athletics. Getting involved in a team sport like soccer, a solo competitive sport like tennis, or something just plain fun like hiking or surfing is an awesome way to get your sweat on. The best part is, you will actually *like* doing it, and you will keep at it for a much longer time than you would continue with that boring old gym routine or mind-numbing cardio machine.

I'm so fat, I look ridiculous working out. I'm so embarrassed.

I know it can be embarrassing to see these fit people exercising and think, "*What am I doing here?*" The answer: you're working on becoming one of the fit people! Instead of thinking, "*I'm so fat,*" just recognize that you *are* taking the steps required to get fit. You are being brave. You are being responsible. You previously let yourself slip, but now you're taking charge. When you think about it, you're virtually a hero!

Also, I'm pretty sure the opposite of your fears is what will actually happen: many people are going to mention to you how much they admire you for what you are accomplishing. Ignore any snickering. One day, you're going to have the last laugh, as others start asking YOU for fitness advice. And seriously, if others actually mock you for putting in the effort to better yourself, they are the ones who should be embarrassed, not you.

8 | October: Learning to Fly

I was finally up to speed. But was I ready to take to the skies?

Friday, Oct 1

12:42 pm – Seven-Day Challenge going well

I feel pretty confident that my ten-day plateau is over! I have lost weight each of the past three days, to the tune of two pounds. I don't know how much of that is because my plateau ended and how much is from the extra self-control ... but I'm not going to ruin things by asking too many questions.

Also, I'm happy to report that I can *feel* my collarbones and hipbones better, even though I can't really *see* them yet. Someday soon, I will.

8:35 pm – Feeling a little high on life

Today I realized I have been swimming a whole kilometer each time I've been out ... and it made me start thinking, *"Isn't that about how far they swim in a triathlon?"*

I looked it up, and it's actually MORE than they swim in a sprint-length triathlon, and 2/3 of what they swim in the Olympic version.

I really must be on drugs, because I am now seriously considering trying a triathlon! How's this sound: 750m swim, 20km bike, 5km run. That's roughly a half mile swim, 12-mile bike, and 3-mile run.

I can barely imagine how cool it would be to say I've done a *triathlon*!

Saturday, Oct 2

10:10 am – Run?

I had a small breakfast half an hour ago. It was raining, but the rain just stopped. Time to whip out my phone, plug in some headphones, start blasting some tunes, and see if I can actually run 5K—since my real 5K race is only three weeks away.

10:15 am – Rain

Okay, the rain started pouring the moment I finished typing my last sentence.
Ugh.
I'M GOING ANYWAY, HAHA!

12:15 pm – Rainrunning

I'm so glad I chose to run! I had a super long run, and the rain stopped after only five minutes. It was ultra-pretty outside, and there was a general lack of people, due to the rain. Win!

All told, I ran 3.3 miles. I have run that far only like three times in my entire life! It feels so good that I have come such a long way. I had to walk for a couple of moments, but I'm pretty sure that in three weeks I will be able to run the entire 5K race. I'm going to aim for a no-walk 5K, which will be a lifetime first if I can pull it off.

9:30 pm – Favorite food?

I just realized I no longer have a favorite food—because I'm simply not beholden to *any* particular foods until I get skinny.

This is obviously the new me talking.

10:25 pm – New record

Tomorrow will be the first time in my life I've exercised SEVEN days in a row! And not just light exercise! Three hard swims, two hard runs, one medium run and one medium elliptical session. All this from someone who used to think that three days of working out in a week was serious exercise!

Monday, Oct 4

10:15 am – Seven-Day Challenge results are IN

I did it!—"it" being seven days of excellent self-control, made possible by going on the Challenge! I just BARELY made it, with no points to spare, at 500 (the minimum required to "succeed") of a possible 560 points.

- Mon: -10: not enough sleep
- Tue: -5: run was a little on the short side
- Wed: -10: too little sleep again
- Thu: -5: exercise was only medium intensity, not hard; also -10 points for eating too much
- Fri: -10: still not getting enough sleep
- Sat: no penalty: good day!
- Sun: -10: food (party—but I ate only a little bit too much)

And the results? Over three pounds lost, and a definite increase in muscle at the same time! Considering I was still on a plateau the first two days of the challenge, I am happy with this, even though it's not the four or five pounds I would have liked to lose.

Now, my thirteen-week summary:

This week was … excellent! For the first time in my life, I am *enjoying* exercise (I always thought others who said the same were *nuts!*). I finally busted through my *ten-day* plateau (sonofabiatch!), and several people commented on how good I look!

Best of all, today marks *20 pounds lost!* One more pound, and I will be halfway there! It has been taking longer than I wanted it to (I know some girls have lost 20 pounds in a single month), but that hasn't stopped me from being *ecstatic* about getting skinny!

2:40 pm – Cutting (ish)

Oh wow … I just saw a picture. It was so crazy. A girl was pinching her stomach fat in one hand, and in the other hand she held a pair of scissors, poised as if to shear off her flab.

This stirs up some crazy memories for me … so many times throughout my life I have wished I could seriously take a knife and just carve my fat off of me ...

Whew, such intense emotions, it's making me dizzy just thinking about it.

Being fat is such a small thing, yet such a huge thing at the same time. I'm so grateful to have found a better way.

6:50 pm – Sad tonight

A couple of crappy things happened today at school. One affects my grade a fair amount, and the other just made me feel like I suck and everyone else is having an easier time than I am. I am feeling very low and just want to go to bed—but I have to study tonight for about four hours.

Yet today started out amazing—and I was the lightest I've been in almost three years.

I guess getting skinny can only go so far in making a person happy.

Tuesday, Oct 5

2:40 pm – Taking tonight off!

Class was cancelled this afternoon! I feel like I need a break, as I'm still in recovery from the Seven-Day Challenge. I've had about 600 calories and it's only 2:30 in the afternoon, but that's okay. I'll probably hit 1000 or even 1200 today (I am sipping on a delicious drink right now, hee hee) but sometimes you just need to let yourself go. BUT, the difference between what tonight will be and what it would have been in the past is:

- *In the past*: four drinks, half a pizza, and ice cream ... then maybe more ice cream ... and maybe one last slice of pizza.
- *Tonight*: two or three drinks, snacking a little bit, but still being smart about it and eating my vegetables.

Haha, with my life now habitually under control, even the "splurge" moments are way less wild than they were before—but it still feels like splurging! I love this.

10:30 pm – I have a dream

I have this fantasy that when I get skinny, I will feel my skin tight on my body wherever I go. When I walk, I will feel the skin stretching over my hipbones. When I swing my arms, I'll feel my shoulder blades sweeping back and forth. When I raise my arms above my head, I'll feel my stomach getting tight and my back muscles rippling under my taut skin.

Whether this is true or not, this fantasy does it for me.

I *will* get skinny.

Wednesday, Oct 6

3:45 pm – Beauty and the gap

Lately, wherever I go, I've been paying more attention to the pretty girls. To my surprise, I have *not* often been noticing thigh gap.

Sure, it's there once in a while, but for the most part, almost nobody has it. I'm convinced that thigh gap is somewhat like collarbones and back dimples: it's a function of genetics more than it is the result of skinny. We can be skinny and beautiful and still have our thighs touch. I would even go so far as to say *most* beautiful women's thighs touch. That's what I've been noticing, anyway.

It's fine to lose weight, but it's important to stay realistic.

4:15 pm – What I didn't do last summer

Last summer, when I flew home to visit family, I was so excited to call up friends I hadn't seen in ages and get together with them.

But I didn't. They never even knew I was in town. Because I was too ashamed to let them see me so fat.

I'm going to cry right now. Oh! How I allowed my lack of self-control to cripple me. Oh, how it also cheated others.

5:00 pm – About to stop hiding on facebook

Another way my fat has affected my life is that I haven't put any recent pics of myself on facebook for years. I even untagged myself from any picture any friend posted where I was in it.

Also, I always felt a little scared each time I would "friend" people I'd only recently met. I feared they would think I was a fraud when they went on my page and looked at my pictures, which were all from when I was skinnier.

This silliness is soon going to stop. Not because I'm going to come clean, but because I'll soon be at a weight where I'm proud to show myself off instead of being mortified to have anyone see how I look.

This is just another reward that I never thought of before beginning this journey. This skinny business is seriously cool.

Thursday, Oct 7

7:40 am – Quasi bipolar

If I didn't record my weight on a graph, I think I'd appear quite bipolar. Yesterday morning, I was all giddy because I'd lost more weight than I had expected to. Yay, me! Today, I jumped on the scale and found all the weight I'd lost. Crap. I am seriously bummed.

The great help in times like this is that I've been making a graph of my weight. There have been many ups, downs, and even long flats from plateaus. The important thing is, given time, the line on the graph has reflected a constant downward trend, despite all the bumps in the road. This has been the key to me keeping my sanity.

8:00 am – My exit plan

A friend asked how I am planning to make changes once I hit my goal. She figured I would just gain all the weight back. I answered: when I do reach my goal weight, it's not going to be much of an issue, as I am not going to return to eating the way I formerly did. I no longer use food as recreation, so I'm not planning to run back to it once I hit my goal. When I get there, I will simply increase my intake to a level appropriate for my weight. If I notice I'm gaining, I'll cut back until I'm back at the weight I want. If I notice I'm getting too skinny (unlikely!), I'll eat more.

I'm pretty sure I've got this figured out. It gives me such lovely confidence.

1:15 pm – Too much

I ate too much at lunch today. I'm going for a run.

This is so much better than the old days, when I would've just hated myself and felt like curling up in a ball.

7:50 pm – Craving exercise instead of food?

Another entry in the "I can't believe this is happening to me" saga: yesterday, when I jumped in the pool, it had been four days since I had been swimming, and the weirdest thing was, *it felt so good* to be exercising again! And not just in a philosophical sense, either, like feeling some sort of relief from guilt. Instead, because my body had been feeling OFF from not exercising for a few days, I actually felt *better* exercising than I had felt sitting around.

This is so weird and new. I am *not* athletic in the least, I am a total klutz who can't do a dance move to save her life. I also am not "returning" to an active lifestyle, because I never *had* an active lifestyle. I grew up reading books and watching TV, not being active. And yet I am feeling some kind of *need* for exercise. What is happening to me?

Saturday, October 9

9:40 am – LML

It's about time! This morning, I am finally HALF. WAY. THERE. Half way from fatty to hottie. Half way from hate my life to love my life. Today, at least, I definitely Love My Life.

1:00 pm – 5K Rehearsal

I decided to try to run 5K, non-stop, in preparation for the race. Prior to today's run, I'd never run 5K without stopping. After today's run … I've still never done it. Sigh.

For some reason, today it was just so hard to run. No idea why. But I didn't cut the distance short. I stopped to walk a few times, but I completed the entire distance, so at least I have one thing to be happy about: I'm not a quitter.

Not anymore.

2:50 pm – 5K time? What time?

A runner friend asked me what my 5K time is. What exactly is a "time" anyway? That's what real runners talk about, and I'm far from being one of those.

I entered this race only to give me a goal to work towards. My goal is to finish in under half an hour. That's a pretty borderline goal, as it would require me to run the whole distance without stopping once. I'm still going to try. I hope having a crowd of spectators will give me the strength to push myself.

I also hope I don't throw up after.

Monday, Oct 11

6:30 pm – Meh

The other night, I was at a special occasion where we celebrated with food. I didn't binge, but I allowed myself to enjoy myself. Well, yesterday I awoke hungry and, again, I ate too much throughout the day. I didn't go to bed hungry like I should have. And then today, I was completely on track to be awesome, but there was a school event with free food. I heaped a ton of salad on my plate, which was good, but I also ate a small serving of pasta and had a small dessert. Total for today was probably 1200 calories. Not what I wanted.

I didn't binge, but I also didn't have my usual self control. It's like, after I hit my half-way point a couple of days ago, I felt like I had arrived or something, and I didn't need to work so hard. That is so untrue; I still have a ton to lose.

I need to remind myself that *this takes work*. I didn't start losing weight by taking the easy path, and I'm not going to lose weight if I now choose that path. I need once again to embrace that empty feeling in my stomach, to not eat until I need to eat, to not let myself have dessert unless I've already been really good all day.

Being ahead in the race isn't enough. I need to actually cross the finish line.

Tuesday, Oct 12

6:25 am – Time to do this right

After three days of *meh*, I'm back on track. I will do this.

Wednesday Oct 13

4:50 pm – Better

Yesterday I finally ate well and lost the better part of a pound. This morning I swam and am set to eat well again. This is more like it. It feels so good to be doing the right thing.

7:50 pm – "A little"

I was thinking about goals, planning to stop at a "pretty good" weight. But then I asked myself, *"Why stop there?"* The difference between "pretty good" and "awesome" is actually quite little—a "little" more self-control for a "little" bit longer.

Thursday, Oct 14

12:25 pm – Sweet compliment!

A classmate said to me today, "Are you a model?" I totally had NO idea what she was talking about! I looked myself up and down to see if she was referring to something unusual about my outfit. Inside, I was like, *WTH?!?* I was wearing semi-nice clothes, but nothing special.

Puzzled, I asked, "What do you mean? Is that a veiled compliment?"

She replied, "It's not veiled."

!!!

It took me several moments to realize that she had given me a compliment because she genuinely thought I looked great. That simply doesn't *happen* to me! It is hard to wrap my head around the idea, but … *I must actually be starting to look good!*

Friday, October 15

11:30 am – Wish

I wish I was someone who stopped eating when depressed, instead of wanting to binge when I'm down. I envy such people.

12:34 pm – Another wish

It's 12:34—time to make a wish!

...

Nope, still fat ...

Saturday, October 16

11:40 pm – 5K approaches

Only one week until the 5K. Tried again today to run the whole distance without stopping. Uhhh ... I'm thinking that my satisfaction on Race Day will be from just finishing, not from finishing without having to walk. I'm starting to be okay with that.

Whatever. Next year I'll own it. Because next year I will weigh nothing.

Sunday, October 17

2:40 pm – VS models

I'm always in awe when I see the Victoria's Secret models in jeans and a simple tee. They look so amazing. Thus proving that skinny looks good in *anything*.

4:15 pm – "Normal" weight

This morning, I was finally below 145! Yikes, that sounds high, but the truth is, it's not that bad: I have spent most of my years between 140-145. It's not a bad weight for me; I don't look all that "fat," but I'm still heavy. It's just that ... oh thank God!!! ... I'm no longer a *gigantic fail fatty!* I am at a weight where I feel fairly "normal".

Wow. I just typed that and it wasn't in my dreams, it was

the truth. After years of being huge, *I'm back to normal.* That is amazing. I kinda want to cry. I thought I was lost forever in fatness, but instead I am back on track. Wow. Wow again. Wow x10 to the *n*th. Wow! *I'm not huge anymore!!!* Crap, I didn't even realize this until just now.

I am so grateful. I really feel like a new person. I thought I was trapped in fatness, but I'm free! I may need some time for this to sink in.

I. Am. No longer. Friggin' fat.

Wow.

I was going to write about other stuff, but I'm too emotional. I have quite a way to go, but at the same time, I've come so far! I never thought it could happen to me.

7:55 pm – *Finally eating a NORMAL amount*

I'm eating a normal amount now! And it's not that I've increased my intake. Rather, it simply feels 100% normal to be eating the small amounts I've been eating. I don't sit there thinking, *"I want to eat more, but I can't or I'll get fat."* Instead, I merely eat small meals, and it feels like the most natural thing in the world. This must be what it's like to be a skinny person!

Of course, there *have* been days when I've had a raging appetite. But EVERY ONE of those days has been the day AFTER I decided to splurge a little. Every time! Moral of the story: bingeing isn't just taking a couple of steps back, it's actually turning around and walking the other way. I must be so careful.

Tuesday, October 19

7:35 am – *Never so happy to be unfashionable*

Today I look slightly silly. Because I'm in my old, out-of-style jeans! These are the jeans I kept in a dark corner of my closet, taking them out every once in a while to try them on and discover how fat I'd become. These are the jeans that made me cry when I thought I would *never* again fit into them because I couldn't figure out how to stop gaining weight.

Today, they're quite comfy.

4:35 pm – Is life fair?

If life was fair, we'd all look like models.

Rather than spending time complaining about this, I'm going to spend my time working out and eating less.

Wednesday, October 20

9:00 am – Waxing poetic

Last night, I was deliriously happy to be losing weight, even to the point of losing sleep over it. I thought to myself, *"Losing weight is such a shallow thing. It's really silly of you to be making such a big deal out of this ... isn't it?"* I wrote this poem as my response:

skinny

getting skinny won't make me
smarter
funnier
nicer
cooler

getting skinny won't get me
truer friends
bluer eyes
higher grades
closer to God

getting skinny won't change the
kindness in my heart
daydreams in my head
talent in my hands
balance in my account

getting skinny won't fix my
remorse over the past
problems in the present
fears about the future
family in any way, ever

getting skinny won't bring
success to my career
meaning to my life
substance to my relationships
contentment to my soul

getting skinny won't cause others to
hearken to what I say
respect the stand I take
appreciate the pain I've known
love me for who I am

but

getting skinny will add years to my life and life to my years
getting skinny will put a song on my lips and a spring in my step
getting skinny will mean I vanquished the foe I never imagined I could defeat
and became the person I never dreamt I could be

that is enough for me

Thursday, Oct 21

10:25 am – Small but lovely surprise

Today, I was leaning against the wall with my hand in my pocket, and I was like, *"What the heck is that slight bulge under my hand?"*

It was my hipbone!

This is new.

Saturday, Oct 23

9:45 pm – T minus ten and counting

My 5K run is in less than ten hours! I'm so nervous. Can I run the whole thing without stopping to walk?

I guess I'll know in about 10.5 hours.

Sunday, Oct 24

2:35 pm – 5K Crazy

I am crazy. I ran the 5K today (details in a moment). How-ever, about an hour ago, I arrived home, still in my running gear. I needed to buy something from the store, so I thought, *"Heck, maybe I'll just run there."*

I ran a whole mile to the store! Yet I had just run a 5K hours earlier! That is a total of over four miles! The best part is, I could have run farther!

I don't like running. I really don't. But I LOVE what it is doing for my body and I LOVE that I am becoming ABLE to do it!

Now, back to the race:

Time: well over my goal of 30 minutes ... sigh.

Walking?: Yes, unfortunately, and on more than one occa-sion. Sadly, I just didn't have the *oomph* today to keep going.

Pace: little kids and old people passed me. Often. But ... I was still ahead of a ton of people. No matter; being one of the slow ones in a race is still faster than being at home on the couch.

Summary: I have completely shrugged off the fact that I had to walk and that my time wasn't awesome. I have come so far since last summer, when I was just a giant lardball who could barely run five minutes. I feel wonderful!

Summary of the summary: races are awesome! The feeling of crossing the finish line with all these people cheering ... it really does feel like an accomplishment. Even if you're the last per-son to finish, everyone there admires you for doing it. And after, you get to casually let it slip in conversation, "Yeah, so while I was running that 5K the other weekend ..."

Next: try one of the following:

1) Another 5K—and this time REALLY PROMISE my-self to not stop at ALL.
2) Run/walk (mostly walk, I'm sure) a half marathon, just to say I've done it.
3) A short (sprint distance) triathlon. Seriously, I can't even imagine how awesome it would be to say that I've done a *triathlon!* I could brag about that every day for a year.

Monday, Oct 25

9:45 am – Reality just wrecked my fantasy

Yeah, so I had several drinks Friday night, more Saturday, and again last night. In my fantasy world, they were just liquids and wouldn't affect my weight.

This morning, I'm fat. I guess I don't have a magically changed body with a faster metabolism after all.

This is so hard some days.

9:00 pm – My new, thin life

Screw my grumbling from earlier. Today is the three-month anniversary of my changed life! If someone had told me before that I was to consistently eat small portions and get regular exercise for three whole months, I would have just scoffed, thinking, *"No way, that's too hard and too long ... I can't do it. I know myself too well. Do you think I haven't already tried?"*

I would have been wrong. So wrong! I've changed, including in how I view food. To my surprise, this hasn't been nearly as hard as I thought it would be—it actually feels rather natural. Sure, I still screw up a little now and then, only now it's the exception, not the rule.

All my life, ALL MY FRIGGIN' LIFE, I've been fat or at least too round. My identity, right down to the core of who I am, was always some version of *fatso.*

But staying on track over the days, weeks, and now months has worked in me a marvelous transformation. I'm not the same person anymore: *I feel skinny now!* I don't mean I actually am; I still have a long way to go. But inside, I know I'm no longer a fatso. I know I can do this, and I know I *will* do it, because I'm a new me. And the new me is skinny.

Thursday, Oct 28

6:30 am – Choosing skinny

I awoke feeling puffy, and the scale confirmed that I was.

Tempted to think: "Screw this, it isn't working! I'm never going to lose the weight, so why bother trying?"

Chose to think: "I ate poorly yesterday, got too little sleep last night, and barely exercised this week. Today, I'm going to wait until I'm genuinely hungry before eating, and then eat only enough to make the hunger subside. I'll go for a long swim this morning and get plenty of sleep tonight."

I can't believe I'm saying all this. It makes me feel so ... *capable*. This is going to work—it has to! My body may try to be a bitch about it, and my head may try to screw with me, but I am going to prevail no matter how long this takes.

The real me is skinny! Body, get used to it! You ARE going to obey your new master.

3:50 pm – Rollin'

I have rolls. I'm looking at them right now.

Time to go for a run. I just want this to be over!

But I guess it's still going to take time. And sweat. And an occasionally growly stomach.

Friday, Oct 29

12:25 pm – Smaller top!

I'm wearing a new top today, and it's more fitted than my other shirts are. Two happy things I've noticed:

1. My posture is way better, because I am standing up straight and sucking in my stomach! If I don't do this, flab shows more than I like.
2. People have really been mentioning how slim I look!

Saturday, Oct 30

4:40 pm – Joyously confused about clothes

It won't be long before "normal fit" clothes are going to look bad on me. I'm not talking about my old clothes (obviously I'll have to get rid of all my fat clothes, yay), but new clothes! I am going to have to start buying brands with a slimmer, tailored fit.

This is such a new, even foreign, idea! It makes me so happy. I have never been skinny before. I've never been able to buy clothes that actually showed off my form.

The funny thing is, I don't even know what brands will look

good on me. It's going to be a completely new shopping experience! This will be so great.

Sunday, Oct 31

8:30 am – [Lack of] Progress Report

I dropped less than a pound this week. That sucks. But it also makes sense: I really wasn't trying very hard.

At least a small loss is better than *any* gain.

1:10 pm – It's time for another Seven-Day Challenge

After my mediocre week, I've decided to go back on the Seven-Day Challenge. Last time, it really helped me to bust through my plateau. This time, I'm not plateauing, but my weight just isn't dropping fast enough. I'm at 142.5 today. I want to be in the 130s by next Sunday.

So far today, I'm only at 375 calories, and it's already afternoon, so I look to be on track. I wasn't going to exercise today, but now I want to go for a run and get this started. If I drink plenty of water and get to bed at a good time, *voilà!* One day down.

I both started and ended the month with my ludicrous, impatience-driven Seven-Day Challenge. Although by this time I had fully spread my wings, any soaring I was doing was merely because I was high on excitement. Fortunately, the lessons would keep coming in, teaching me what it took to safely stay aloft.

Q&A | On Eating Disorders

Skinny is satisfying—but skinny alone can never satisfy.

People wonder if I'm "pro-ana," meaning that I encourage anorexia. Seeing as I portray hunger in a positive light, this comes as no surprise.

I'm certainly *not* "pro-ana" in the sense that I encourage people to behave like anorexics. On the contrary, I am against starving yourself or purging, and I would caution against *anything* excessive or extreme when it comes to weight loss, even excessive exercise.

However, I *am pro* ("for") the *people* who suffer from anorexia and other EDs. I am sad that they are so unhappy and in the grip of such dangerous thinking and habits. I would never revile nor condemn them. I wish them only the best, and I pray they figure out how to win their war. That's the only acceptable way to be "pro-ana," as far as I know.

However, because we're on the subject, let's take a brief look at EDs, beginning with discovering what eating disorders actually consist of. Specifically, let's look at Anorexia, Bulimia, Binge Eating Disorder, and EDNOS / FEDNEC.

ANOREXIA

The official name of this disorder is Anorexia Nervosa, and it requires ALL of the following:

1. you restrict your intake to the point that you become underweight;
2. you intensely fear gaining weight or becoming fat (or if "fear" isn't the word, you still try to interfere with weight gain) even though you're at a significantly low weight; and

3. you think you're fatter than you are / you give your weight or shape too great of an influence in how you feel about yourself / you dismiss the importance of maintaining a healthy weight in favor of obtaining a super low weight.

Anorexia gets sub-classified even further, because not all anorexics use the same methods. There are the "Restricting Type," who do merely eat too little, and the "Binge Eating / Purging Type," who engage in regular bingeing or purging—which is NOT limited to throwing up, but also includes using laxatives, enemas, or diuretics—to lower the number on the scale.

BULIMIA

Officially called "Bulimia Nervosa". It requires (again, ALL must be present):

1. a pattern of bingeing, meaning you eat way more over a certain period of time (even if it takes a couple of hours of continued snacking) than most people would eat in that time, and while you're bingeing, you feel like you can't control your eating;
2. you make up for these binges with purging, fasting, using laxatives/diuretics, or excessively exercising;
3. you've been doing this about once a week or more for at least the last three months; and
4. you give your weight or shape too great an influence in how you feel about yourself.

BINGE EATING DISORDER

This one describes those who binge—and hate themselves because of it—but don't engage in compensatory behavior like purging, fasting, or extreme exercise. It requires:

1. a pattern of bingeing (same definition as above, and you're doing it about once a week or more for at least the last three months); and
2. you find yourself doing three or more of the following when you binge:
   - scarfing down your food way too fast;
   - eating so much you wind up uncomfortably full;

- eating a ton when you're not even hungry;
- hiding your eating because you're embarrassed by how much it is; or
- feeling depressed / embarrassed / disgusted with yourself for your overeating.

FEEDING / EATING DISORDER NOT ELSEWHERE CLASSIFIED

This replaces what was formerly called EDNOS (Eating Disorder Not Otherwise Specified). I'm calling it FEDNEC until someone comes up with something better. It's proof that letting *anything* about your eating get out of hand is a problem that may need clinical intervention. It comes into effect if ANY (it doesn't require all) of the following are present with enough of an effect that it starts to mess with your life and happiness:

- you have all of the symptoms of Anorexia, but you're not underweight;
- you have all of the symptoms of Bulimia or Binge Eating Disorder, but you don't act out quite frequently enough to qualify;
- you don't meet the qualifications for a "regular" ED, but you tend to use purging as a method to get skinny;
- you frequently eat after your evening meal, even though you realize you shouldn't, and it severely gets you down; or
- your eating habits meet no definition of any of the above, but they still interfere seriously with your life and happiness.

So. Now you have the most up-to-date definitions of the official eating disorders. Before we go on, I need to stop and tell you something. Writing this section has been incredibly *weird* and hard for me to do. The only reason I'm including it is to ALERT you to the fact that you may have a legitimate weakness. Yet I feel so creepy typing it all out, because it feels like I'm offering you a *menu* of choices. Not so! PLEASE recognize that ALL OF THESE THINGS RUIN YOUR LIFE!!! This is NOT a fad you get into. It's not a label you attach to yourself to achieve some kind of club status. THESE THINGS KILL. And even if they don't prove fatal or ruin your health, they will kill you on the inside. You are far too lovely to allow something like this to take away your joy and health. PLEASE don't. If you see yourself depicted in any of the above descriptions, you NEED to seek help (seeking help is a sign of strength, not weakness—it means you are able to do the right thing even when it's uncomfortable). Putting it off will only make things worse and make you both unhappier and unhealthier.

At school, I can skip lunch without my parents finding out, but at home, I'm forced to eat. Later, I find it difficult to throw up. How can I lose the weight?

As warmly and as friendlily as I can, allow me to say:
1. *Small* meals, *not* skipped meals.
2. No purging.
3. Determination, not desperation.

I exercise all the time. I was recently told I might have "exercise bulimia". I'm confused: how is exercise a bad thing?

If you really do have exercise bulimia, the problem is not the exercise (or else professional athletes, who exercise for hours every day, would all have exercise bulimia). The problem is WHY you exercise.

Typically, people with exercise bulimia feel the need to either (a) punish themselves for their eating; or (b) go to extremes to achieve a goal … extremes they can't keep up forever and which will later lead to greater feelings of failure. The most ironic thing about exercise bulimia is that others, meaning well, will applaud the bulimic person, not realizing she is destroying herself, because exercise is usually counted a good thing.

The problem rests in the unhealthy, self-critical attitude *behind* the exercise. It is destructive. If the description above (self-flagellation or extreme devotion) describes how you feel, you may well have an ED, and you might actually be in danger of being destroyed. Destroyed by a black hole of regret and self-loathing. It's a deadly trap.

If, on the other hand, this isn't you, please count yourself blessed, and watch that it doesn't come to this. Because Exercise Bulimia is like poison disguised as medicine.

I used to be fat, but now I'm 30 pounds underweight. I know it sounds crazy, but losing that weight is the only thing I've done that I'm proud of.

My dear, I'm happy for you that you were able to cease being overweight. I'm also saddened that you really have taken this so far. I can understand how much happier you are to be skinny now, but I'd be very surprised if you don't still dislike or even hate your body on the deepest level, perhaps so deep you can't even see it yourself. No body you can obtain, nor any praise from others, will ever be perfect enough to heal you of what's hurting you.

No matter what you weigh on the outside, there is a lovely and loveable person on the inside. You are worth much. I myself have experienced much pain from feeling worthless, shameful, self-critical, depressed, you name it. I've also found healing for most of that pain. Much of the pain was from self-inflicted injuries, and I just needed to stop beating myself up. Some of it required me to forgive others. I also needed, and often do need, forgiveness. When I've dealt with these things, I find myself at peace. It's an amazing place. You can get there, too.

Formerly, I merely disliked my body. Anorexia seemed like the most convenient answer. Lately, however, I've come to really hate my body. I hate even more that I love being hungry. I hate when I can feel my food turning straight into fat. I hate everything. I wish I'd never started, but I can't stop. I can't do this anymore. I'm so disgusting. I wish I could just die.

You sweet thing, for real, this is not about fat or skinny. This is about you. You have an unrealistic view of yourself, and about how food works. In many ways, it's not your fault. You need to figure out what's going on behind the scenes. I honestly recommend finding a good, friendly, professional therapist and explaining things to her. I know it sounds intimidating, or embarrassing, or even creepy. But sometimes the right professional can help you understand yourself so much better than anyone else ever could.

I also recommend you take it up in prayer. Not just *"Help me!"* prayer, but *"I want to know what's real, and I want to really figure things out and set things right"* prayer. That's the way to obtain the most powerful answers.

I don't have an ED, but I find myself drawn to the idea, especially when I visit some of the pro ana blogs.

So you've found the darker side of the weight loss community. To go online and look for inspiration is to stumble upon some of these sites. If your head is in a certain place, such sites can seem attractive, intriguing, even romantic. You might feel like your life is boring in comparison, and like you have nothing special about yourself to take pride in. In times like this, you might actually take comfort in acquiring an eating disorder. That way, you at least have a Label. You finally belong to a Group. A Secret Society. The odd thing is, even though you know it's a dangerous group to belong to, you're still just too fascinated to let go of the idea. Of course you're careful about things. You're not about to dive right in, so you merely dip your toe in the water. Yet even that takes a lot of self-control, so you're tempted to become proud of your accomplishment because, hey, not everyone can be this strong!

That's not strength, that's weakness. That's permitting something else to have power over you. But you won't see it that way, because you're too excited to be part of this exciting underground cult that makes its members feel so tragically beautiful.

Next thing you know, you find that you really have cast yourself into those dark waters. You'll be adrift in them. Except, by then, you'll be even more strengthened in your resolve, because now it's not a fault, it's just who you are. It's how you're wired. It's your "ED". You're not the *perpetrator*, you're the *victim*. Victims' problems are not their fault. Victims deserve sympathy. Suddenly, it's not your choices that caused you to sink into this spot, it's society's fault, it's your parents' fault, it's anybody's fault but yours. You will come to actually believe this lie, even though it's a lie you will have told yourself.

It's hard to arrive in a worse place than to be ensnared in this kind of downward spiral. Others can't pull you out, you aren't willing to pull yourself out, and you won't even want to reach out for help because it's just easier to retreat into this nightmare you created for yourself and to commiserate with the other lost souls trapped in the same dark dream. Even though it's a nightmare, you'll want to remain there, because others can't hurt you there.

Except that's not true. Others can and will hurt you plenty, only you won't fully recognize it, because you'll be too numb from the pain you're already inflicting upon yourself. You will be, in effect, trapped. In darkness. With your only chance for survival being the abandonment of all you have embraced—yet you're too afraid to let go.

You can do better than that. That isn't you. That's not the real you. The real you is lovely—perhaps hidden at this moment, but definitely lovely. Take those courageous steps that will lead you to discovering the real you.

CONCLUSION

I need to draw this chapter to a close. I wish I could go on and on for pages. There is so much deliverance to be found! You needn't be a slave to your passions. You needn't hate yourself. But this isn't a book on EDs, so I have to move on. Just remember: *lack of fat does not equal satisfaction with self.* Yes, it hurts to have unwanted fat, but, regardless of your weight, it hurts even more to disapprove of who you are.

If you simply follow the advice in this book—and I *don't* mean just the "it's okay to be hungry" advice—you will be living a healthy life of self-control, reaping both instant and permanent rewards. If, however, you find yourself focusing on your fat, or on severe restricting, or on constant exercising, or even on your guilt for overeating—you REALLY need to be careful! My motto is "Thin *gives* life," not "Thin *is* life"! Get it wrong, and you're in serious trouble. If you suspect I'm talking directly to you, PLEASE seek real help outside these pages.

There *are* steps you can take that lead to thin and happy without causing you harm and misery. Your life doesn't have to be a disaster. Consider, for example, the following message I received from someone who figured it out: *"Today at lunchtime, I ate more than I should have eaten. I was going to purge it, but I just didn't want to continue the cycle of negativity. Instead, I skipped the bus and walked home from school. I didn't burn all of the extra calories, but I don't care because I know this is the start of a healthier me."*

Guess what? Today can also be the start of a healthier you.

10 | November: Hitting my Stride

Having ironed out the major wrinkles, I found myself making major progress. Good habits were easier to maintain, and I suffered fewer setbacks. Many people began to notice the changes in me. Happily, I was one of those people.

Monday, Nov 1

10:35 am – Annoying "friend" episode

I used to be fatter than a really good friend at school. I'm now skinnier than she is. She's obviously impressed that I lost weight, but now she's telling me to stop, because this "weight looks really good" on me, "I shouldn't lose any more," etc ...

This annoys me so much! If I start getting close to the "underweight" portion of the chart, *then* you've got a point, but not before.

Wednesday, Nov 3

9:35 am – Are my goals valid?

I was pondering the legitimacy of my goal again. Is it really important that I work until I reach perfection? Isn't that a silly, unobtainable goal?

Except I don't seek perfection. I just want to fix what's broken. I don't need to be better than others, I just want to be better than me. It's different. And it's a valid goal.

10:00 am – Four days into the Seven-Day Challenge

Swam today for 40 minutes, making it the fourth day in a row that I've gotten good exercise. I exceeded the permitted number of calories, but still kept it reasonable. Water and sleep not a problem. The stage today looks set for success.

After three days, I've lost a pound. I need to lose one and a half more by Sunday morning. That means I will be into the 130s, and will be less than ten pounds away from setting a *new record low weight!*

Thursday, Nov 4

7:15 am – My plan

Plan for today: go to bed healthier than I awoke.

3:00 pm – Running was all the way easy!

Wow, I went for a run and, I swear, I was barely breathing heavily! The weather was warm, which usually gives me energy, but I think the main reason my run was easy is that *I am skinnier than I used to be!*

I swear I could feel the difference. I don't have as much flab swinging around anymore. Even my feet could feel how much lighter I weigh; instead of *thudding* onto the pavement, I was more *padding* along.

Happy!

Friday, Nov 5

6:30 am – Two more days to lose one more pound

If I lose another pound, the Seven-Day Challenge will have worked and gotten me into the 130s.

And if I don't, it doesn't matter, because I will be there soon enough.

This morning, I'm so happy to be getting skinny! So profoundly happy.

Saturday, Nov 6

8:30 am – Thinspo need dissipating

I've been noticing that I don't "need" thinspo like I used to. Thinspo used to be my primary weight loss motivator when I felt trapped in my body and wanted to give up. Now that I've lost weight and am daily enjoying the benefits from doing so, I've changed and I don't really need so much thinspo. Instead:

- I know I *can* do it.
- I know it's a lifestyle I can endure and even *enjoy*.
- I know that *the real me, the skinny me, is poised to emerge.*

Thinspo or no thinspo, I'm never going back.

6:40 pm – New Record!

I can't believe it. I set a new world record today! Well, my world, anyway.

I went for a run with no idea how far I would go; I just knew I wanted to go farther than usual to make up for eating too much last night.

I ran for a freaking HOUR! I covered over five miles! This shatters my previous record!

This is *so* big! I remember how excited I was, months ago, the day I was able to run for ten minutes before stopping to walk and catch my breath. I thought that was about as good as I was going to get. Today, however, after pausing to walk a few times, I realized *I didn't even need to stop.*

It used to be that every time I ran, every extra minute of running got harder and harder, until I was too out of breath to continue. Today, I was just chugging along, breathing heavily, but I somehow seemed to *stabilize* or something, where my running stayed at the same level of difficulty, without getting harder. In the final 22 minutes of my HOUR of running, I didn't stop to walk at all, because I realized I could just keep going! In fact, the only reason I stopped after an hour is because one hour seemed like a nice, round number.

This is unreal. I always thought that even though *other people* can exercise, it would always be different for *me*. Too hard, I'm not built for it, etcetera, etcetera … I have been WRONG the whole time. *I can do this after all!* I've never been so happy to be wrong.

Waves of joy and relief are flooding over me. I didn't know this was possible. Not for me.

I guess I'm no longer the "me" I thought I was.

Sunday, Nov 7

2:00 pm – Seven-Day Challenge results

So close! I almost lost the 2.5 pounds required to bust me into the 130s. Instead, I lost only 2.2. No matter, it was still a success, and I am now *officially within ten pounds of setting a new record low weight!* I guess losing 2.2 lbs in only a week is actually quite good, so I shouldn't complain.

On a side note, my fitness app says I burned almost 3000 calories in exercise in the past week. I read somewhere that 3500 calories equals one pound of fat. My fat's days are numbered.

If I continue with perfect behavior (unlikely), I will hit 125 by Christmas. A more likely result is that I will hit 125 sometime in January. I'll take it!

Tuesday, Nov 9

11:00 am – Close call with an apple fritter

Wow, that was close. I was offered my choice of a free doughnut and, sitting there in the box mocking me, was an apple fritter—my favorite kind! I actually decided to go for it. BUT thankfully that decision lasted only about a second, or the time it took me to remember that eating that sucker would screw me to the tune of about 600 – 700 calories.

I'm still craving a bite of sweet, soft, apple-y fritter. But I'm enjoying the sweet savor of victory even more.

Thursday, Nov 11

8:30 am – Sadness/loathing

I've been thinking. Every day, I drive past a billboard advertising a stomach-altering procedure that makes it harder for people to eat large meals. It costs something like $50,000. And it involves dangerous surgery.

Sadness: people don't need this! We just need to learn self-control! With self-control comes the joy of victory instead of the pain of slavery to our passions.

Loathing: our culture is just so out of control! We live lives of excess and exhibit virtually no accountability for behavior. So many people want an instant fix, and they want someone else to fix things for them.

Is there any hope?

10:20 am – "Short" run?

I just ran over a mile and a half, without stopping, and thought of it as a "short" run. I was barely even breathing heavily. What is happening to me?

Friday, Nov 12

3:20 pm – Going for a new record tomorrow

Tomorrow, weather permitting, I'm going to try to best the record I set last week. I'm going to see if I can do 6.55 miles, which would be a quarter of a marathon. That would pretty much make my week.

I'm also so excited, thinking of how much easier running will be once I get down to my Goal Weight!

Saturday, Nov 13

7:45 am – Grrrr

I took it easy the past week. I lost zero pounds. There's no easy way to lose weight.

1:05 pm – 1/4 marathon!

I did it! And this time, I walked LESS in 6.55 miles than I walked in last week's 5.1 miles—because I've learned that I don't HAVE to walk nearly as much as I thought I did! In fact, today, in 75 minutes of running, I took only four short walking breaks!

I'm not even all that close to my goal weight, and yet I've changed so much. I'm basically a different person.

- I'm no longer hugely fat.
- I'm no longer a slave to my appetite.
- I no longer fit into any of my old clothes.
- I no longer think I can't do it—whatever "it" is.

- I now realize that my own choices make a greater difference than my surrounding circumstances do. This is such a total flip-flop from my old way of thinking.
- I wish I could hug everyone in the world and tell them, *YOU, TOO, CAN DO IT!*

Monday, Nov 15

11:30 am – Hello 130s!

Yes!!! This morning I finally just squeaked into the 130s, at 139.8!

Gosh that number still sounds so high ... but it is a FAR CRY from my (ugh!) starting weight.

I have fewer than 15 pounds to go. I am 2/3 of the way to my goal. I'm no longer fat, I'm merely flabby. I'm going to make it, I know it!

Tuesday, Nov 16

11:00 am – Butterflies

My heart literally flutters when I think of how awesome it will feel to be skinny. It's like I have a crush on my future self.

11:20 am – On ducks and swans

When I first started this adventure, I paid close attention to who noticed my weight loss. Some weeks, nobody noticed. I was so excited the week that *three* people mentioned that I was looking good.

Well, today, it's not even lunchtime, and already three people have complimented me on my looks, including one [gorgeous] classmate who said that "you can really tell" I've slimmed down. I don't mean to be vain, but THIS FEELS AMAZING!

Even strangers of both sexes are treating me better and are friendlier. And I'm still not even skinny yet! This just rocks SO MUCH.

Is it possible that I'm actually a swan after all, and not just an ugly duckling???

Wednesday, Nov 17

8:50 pm – Odd method of appetite suppression

Tonight, I was really grumpy and stressed out and I just wanted to stuff my face, but I was at school and had no food. I went for a swim instead. Appetite gone, energy back, mood elevated! One of the nicest surprises I've had in ages.

Sunday, Nov 21

2:40 pm – Well this isn't working

The past two weeks, I've just been assuming that the weight is going to keep falling off of me, but it hasn't changed. I'm pretty sure that the problem is that I've been too lazy with the portion control.

Sooooo ...

So I'm going to count calories for a week, just to re-teach myself what a day's food intake is supposed to look like. I'm also going to post each day's intake online. If I don't post it, I'm more prone to cheat. When I know I have to admit it in public, it helps me to think twice before stuffing my face.

6:50 pm – Intake

800 calories so far. I promise not to eat any more tonight. So, today looks like a success. Hope the scale agrees with me tomorrow.

10:05 pm – Unexpected bonus

I don't know whether it's the swimming or the running (or both, duh) that I have to thank, but my butt is really shaping up. Of course it's getting skinnier, but it's also a lot shapelier. I totally have muscles that I can flex back there. My side profile is not nearly as flat as it used to be.

This is alright!

Wednesday, Nov 24

8:20 am – Rant

I'm still quite chubby in a lot of places. Not overly-critical with myself, not skewed by an ED, just legitimately chubby. But I've been getting a lot of flak from others because I want to continue losing weight.

And yet I'm sure that NOBODY would choose to have my body over a healthy, thin body, if it were up to them.

People keep pointing me to websites where overweight girls talk about how they have accepted their overweight bodies, and are proud of them, and go on about how beautiful they are. "Proud to have curves" I can handle; some of us are just built that way. Proud to be overweight is different: it means you're proud of failure. Count me out.

9:15 am – Enough whining already

Good news: I awoke 3/4 of a pound lighter today!

The past three days, I dropped only a tiny bit of weight, but today was a really nice surprise. When I awoke, I even felt skinnier. Lying in bed, running my hands over my tummy, I was able to feel my ribs poking out not just at the prominent peaks on the sides but also near the top where they come together (my sternum?). Hipbones are also coming along.

This, after a two-week plateau, is most welcome!

Counting calories appears to be working. I guess I had been getting more food than I realized I was getting, by not paying enough attention. Note to self.

3:15 pm – Serendipitous success

Sitting around the house. Had the day off. Decided to go for a long scenic run. Ran 8.5 miles, another gigantic shattering of my previous record!

8:50 pm – OMG jeans win!

I am down a size! I picked up a pair of gorgeous—no, make that *GORGEOUS*—designer jeans for cheap at a rack store. They are so well made, it's just amazing. I could just stroke them, they feel so soft. They are tight on me, but I know they won't be for long.

Gosh, it feels good to be wearing these jeans. My old jeans were getting baggy (a nice problem to have!), but these new jeans hug my hips really tight. When I walk along, instead of just sorta *moving*, I can feel my hips *swaying*. It's hard to describe, but it's wonderful. I have a ton of confidence in my new jeans. And since they fit a little tight, they should soon fit perfectly as I keep losing weight.

I also bought another amazing pair of jeans, for $100 (down from $300). They are another size smaller, so I can't wear them yet, but they are *even more gorgeous!* I bought them as my "Goal Jeans". When I lose another ten pounds or so, I will wear them and just beam the biggest smile ever.

11:05 pm – Going to bed happy

Tomorrow is the four-month anniversary of my new healthy life. I remembered that fact especially sweetly today because, while on my epic run, I ran past the very spot of beach where, at the picnic last July 25, I ate my first responsible meal. I hadn't seen that place since. I ran(!) past it today as a new person in so many ways. I am so thankful. I can't believe this is happening. I am no longer a prisoner of my body. I'm actually starting to quite like my body! Is this a dream? No, it's real.

Add to that the fact that I just weighed myself tonight—and I'm already lighter than I was first thing this morning. That means tomorrow I will awake even lighter! It's all so wonderful!

Thursday, Nov 25

7:25 am – I'm starting off the day on the right foot!

1. It's Thanksgiving.
2. It's the four-month anniversary of my new, healthy life.
3. I dropped over a pound today! I'm 0.2 pounds away from having lost 30.

To celebrate, I'm going to ~~eat enough to sink a ship~~ decide in advance to eat only a tiny amount of Thanksgiving dinner tonight, no matter that it is Thanksgiving. Then I will REALLY make this an awesome day!

Oh, sweet skinny attitude, where have you been all my life?

9:30 am – Meeting the real me

I've had my story[11] posted online for a few weeks. Someone commented that it must have taken a long time to write.

The funny thing is: it didn't. I actually sat down and banged out the whole thing in one go. In a way, I don't even know where it came from.

Today, I figured it out: that was the Real Me talking. Not the "new" me, the *Real Me*.

As I've watched my new, skinny body emerge over the months, and as I've seen my attitude and whole way of thinking change for the better, I've gotten excited, thinking that I'm becoming a "new" person. However, I think what is happening instead is that *the Real Me is finally being allowed to emerge*. The Real Me that was buried all along. Now, with the obscuring fat melting away, and the smothering shame lifted by the buoyancy of my newfound hope, I can finally make out the Real Me.

If this was actually a "new" me arriving, I would be afraid that I wouldn't be able to trust myself, because I wouldn't know what I'm doing. Instead, the Real Me is trustworthy, because it's not an act, and it's not me trying to imitate anybody. It's more me being *myself* for the first time, like I'm a caged bird finally going free. I mean, just because I haven't yet been allowed to fly doesn't mean that flight isn't, to me, the most natural thing in the world.

The real me is confident, gracious, thankful, and lovely. The real me doesn't envy those who look amazing but cries for those who don't. The real me is skinny but doesn't flaunt it.

I am so honored to have recently become acquainted with Real Me. I rest in a breathless, quiet joy that soon, not many pounds from now, she will be revealed to everyone around me. When that happens, I will never again permit her to remain hidden away.

11:05 am – Random thought

I just had a tiny little fantasy which made me smile. I've heard people say this to others before, but now I can look forward to the day when somebody says to *me*, "If you get any

---

[11] What is now Chapter One (minus the graph, which obviously wasn't complete until later).

skinnier, you'll blow away!"

Just remembered an odd and amazing thrill from long ago, when I was at my lowest weight. I had been exercising a lot, and my weight had gotten down somewhat, while my muscle tone was halfway decent. I was in bed on a lazy Saturday morning, lying flat on my tummy. I reached around behind me to arrange my sheets, searching for that perfect amount of coverage to keep me from getting chilly, but not so much coverage that I overheated. Unaware that I had arched my back a tiny bit in order to reach my sheets, I startled myself when my hand brushed against the small of my back. I was like, *"WHAT was that? I think I just felt something sexy!"*

Unbeknownst to me, much of my fat had receded in that area, allowing the contours of my spine, those gorgeous, sexy lower back contours, to surface. On *me!* Un. Real.

I spent a long time, over half an hour, caressing my back and, to be honest, fantasizing. Not fantasizing just about being skinny, but about being able to share those sexy contours with someone who would be excited—even more excited than I was—to enjoy them. It was more than a little bit arousing. I laid in bed luxuriating on a wonderful, dreamy cloud.

That memory faded when I started gaining weight soon after. I hid it in a dusty box of painful memories on a shelf way in the back of my mind, a passing moment of *almost tasting* what it would be like to be sexy.

I accidentally stumbled upon that dusty old box recently. Lately while doing certain things like stretching, tucking my shirt in, showering, or what have you, I've noticed that there is way less give in that area of my back, less padding. My back has been feeling more and more slender, more … tight. The hidden contours are again resurfacing. This has rekindled in me a wonderful feeling. I thought hotness—really, only "near" hotness—was always going to remain just a fantasy. Now I realize that not only near hotness—but *real* hotness—is very near.

That is more than a little bit arousing.

12:30 pm – New rule

I'm about to head out for Thanksgiving dinner, and I'm reminding myself of my new rule: *No more eating it just because it's there.*

May I remember this rule for the rest of my life.

Saturday, Nov 27

1:30 pm – Burger hate

I used to love hamburgers, especially the thick restaurant kind, but I haven't eaten one in months. I don't miss them. Those suckers just made me fat anyway.

On that note, it's time to go for a run. A friend asked me what my 5K time has gotten down to. I didn't know what to tell her, so I'm going to go find out right now!

I love having an incentive to exercise, because sometimes I really need one.

3:00 pm – Cipe

My run was cipe, or epic spelled backwards. It was really hard. It was cold out, so my lungs felt unhappy, plus my legs got tired really quickly. Obviously, something must be way off today, because 5K is no longer a long run for me. Bleh.

My time was well over half an hour, same as the 5K I did last month. I should've been way faster today, but at least I wasn't slower. I'm grumpy about this, but really, if I think about it from the right perspective, today was a triumph. At least I got out there and ran.

7:50 pm – The healthy way

Another reason I know I'm going about this the healthy way is: rather than concentrating on my current flaws, I've been spending more time noticing what I like about my increasingly slender body … and even more time fantasizing about walking around confidently, someday soon, in a truly great body.

Sunday, Nov 28

9:20 am – Skinny: so much more than a number

It just hit me last night: I'm actually going to be skinny.

For the first time in my life, I'm really going to make it, I know I am. I'm already almost there. For the first time, I'm going to know what it's like.

When I get skinny:

- I'll know what it is to do up my pants without my waist bulging.
- I'll wear normal sized clothes, yet they'll still be roomy.
- I'll be firm to the touch, no longer squishy.
- I'll turn my head to the side and reveal the beautiful lines of my neck, without a chubby chin obscuring the view.
- In fact, screw chins, I'll have only one, even when looking downward.
- My thighs won't chafe when I run.
- My stomach won't jiggle when I giggle.
- I'll resist people tickling me because it actually tickles me, not because it shames me.
- Strangers I meet will wait to get to know me instead of promptly dismissing me at first sight.
- At the beach, I'll get a full tan, not just arms and legs.
- At the doctor's office, I'll be applauded, not admonished.
- My driver's license will finally tell the truth about my weight.
- I will stand up straight rather than trying to collapse and hide.
- I will smile at strangers and actually see them smile back.
- I will accept people's compliments instead of negating them with criticism.
- Alone, I will even compliment myself.

Skinny is not just a number. Skinny is rebirth.

Monday, Nov 29

11:10 am – Compliments!

I've been getting compliments every day lately. The new jeans appear to be working!

2:35 pm – Much post-Thanksgiving happiness

A classmate said to me, "You're the only one in the whole school who *lost* weight over Thanksgiving!" It didn't feel bad to hear that!

Also, earlier, I had an interesting moment of male attention. Settling into my seat in class, I walked past a seated classmate and noticed his eyes following me, only they were aimed around the level of my hips, not my face. I know I'm supposed to be bothered by this, but at this stage it's novel enough that I couldn't help but feel a little bit wonderful.

4:15 pm – Doctor weighs in on weight loss

Saw a new doctor today. She asked a ton of questions. When I answered one question by mentioning that I've lost almost 30 pounds since July, she asked, "You mean since July last year?" I told her no, I mean since four months ago. Uh oh! I leaned back and braced for her to jump all over me for losing too much weight too quickly.

Surprise! Instead she told me how awesome that is! She even went off on a little tirade on how bad it is to be fat and how so many health problems in this country are caused by fat and blah blah blah. She actually supported and congratulated me!

That was the most validating thing since … I don't know, it's kind of in a league of its own!

6:50 pm – Appetite suppression

I have a *raging* appetite right now. Not hunger, just a massive, overwhelming appetite. This is still hard sometimes.

Tuesday, Nov 30

7:00 pm – Future dirty secret

Soon I will be skinny, and when I meet people who never knew the fat me, they won't believe I was ever anything but gorgeous. I can't wait!

Losing weight was obviously exciting in tons of surprising ways. Yet there was still so much more to learn. To my surprise, it wasn't all pretty.

Q&A | Making it through Cravings and Plateaus

The object of your cravings will never satisfy you compared to making it through without giving in.

It happens to all of us. There's no way around it. Sooner or later—no, just make that sooner—you are going to have to deal with the torture of cravings and the frustration of plateaus. Cravings you know to expect, and can even plan around them. A plateau, however, is usually a surprise and almost always a substantial blow to your mood and motivation. Here are some tips to deal with each.

CRAVINGS

Cravings. You can't prevent them. Sometimes they are inhumanly bad. In general, to avoid succumbing:

1. Make sure there is NO tempting snack food around. This sucks at times, but not nearly as much as being fat does.
2. Ride it out without bingeing. You will be so happy that you are making progress that your joy will give you strength.
3. Make it a habit to resist, and, with time, it will become natural to say No. It sounds like a fairy tale, but I promise, it's true!
4. Even so, sometimes you find yourself in that place where there's just no way you're not eating that. At these times, it can be okay to give in JUST A LITTLE. Take a nibble, not a serving. You actually enjoy it more when you permit yourself only a little bit. It becomes even better when later you don't hate yourself.

I get serious munchies at nighttime, and can't get away from the house. What to do?

Nighttime is tough. All those people who recommend we eat a big breakfast, a moderate lunch, and a tiny dinner? That's not real life. That's the opposite of how many of us have to battle our cravings. It's also why I eat such tiny amounts throughout the day; I know I'm going to have a hard time preventing myself from eating more in the evening, no matter what.

Something about nighttime eating just feels right. You're bored, you're near the kitchen ... it can really suck. Plus, you're tired, making you give in more easily than at other times. Ironically, if you policed your eating really well during the day, you're tempted to feel like you can relax your self-control and reward yourself. It can be deadly.

What has often gotten me through this hour of temptation is to learn to love the feeling of going to bed a little hungry. I get a real pleasure out of it. It means I'm winning. It feels many times better than satisfying the cravings does, many times better than going to bed full and awaking with the same weight instead of a new low number on the scale.

All I can suggest is: try it. Promise yourself you'll do well tonight, no matter the cost. Rejoice in the feeling of euphoria you have when you finally slip between your bed sheets and you didn't give in. Then see if you can get used to that wonderful feeling of victory on a more regular basis. On the day you reach your goal, you will be so glad you did.

I usually eat well all day but lose it when I arrive home. Lately, I've found myself gorging on [food X] when I get home. What's my problem?

Your problem? You're human!

Each of us has our own Achilles' Heel. For me, for example, it used to be toast. It was so addicting! I'd make two slices, then two more, and before long I'd eaten half a dozen, each with a generous portion of butter and jam. So wrong! It only relented after I got rid of my toaster.

If I were you, I'd get rid of all the [food X] in the house and not buy any more until I've taught myself to have better self-control. Sometimes, it's just too hard to resist, and you need to cast out the offending item. It's a bit drastic, but some of us *need* drastic, at least when we're first starting out.[12]

It started with a single cookie. And then it turned into pizza. I needed neither. I'm so angry with myself!

I've noticed that eating is inertial. Once I start, it's hard to stop. The worst is when I'm in the kitchen and I decide to have just "a bite" of something, but then I keep eating. The best way to prevent this is to plan your meal, make it, then eat it somewhere away from the food source.

Also, I try to consider how great it feels to lose weight compared to how horrible it feels to eat what I don't need. I still screw up from time to time. In moments like that, I just try to look to the future, not to the past.

What should I do in those moments when I know I don't need to eat, but food is the only thing on my mind?

Egad! Cravings!

I sometimes give in to them, actually. We all do. What saves me is that I've gotten so much into the habit of forcing myself to eat only small amounts that even my cravings never turn into binges anymore. With consistent effort and application, you, too, can train yourself to eat well on a regular basis.

Of course, there's more to it. I mean, if you've read this book from the beginning, you've seen some deep stuff going on in my head as I readjust my ways of thinking to adopt a skinny attitude. You, too, need to think some things through. For starters, try thinking of skinny as freedom and cravings as your captor. Ask yourself: do you want to be free?

---

[12] However, I still have no toaster. I know myself too well.

PLATEAUS

Plateaus provide some of the strongest temptations to give up. It looks like your efforts aren't paying off. You question, "Why go through all this discomfort when it doesn't even work?"

Plateaus are where the rubber meets the road. Hitting one is like your first time playing solo in a concert, like taking that brutal college entrance exam, like Game Point when it's your serve. You've already been practicing your weight loss routine, learning about health, and strategizing your meals. You've made real progress, but now comes the time to see what you're really made of. A plateau is not the time to think about giving up. It's time to Bring It.

I'm completely on track. My eating is super strict and I'm exercising hard several times a week. But my weight hasn't budged in days! What's going on?

Sometimes your body is just a bitch. That's a fact. When stuff like this happens to me, I just take comfort in knowing that it CANNOT last! Don't give up. You don't know for certain that sticking with it just a little longer isn't all you need, but you *do* know for certain that giving up can only set you back.

What's your experience with plateaus? How do you overcome one and how long does it take you?

I've had several major plateaus, including times when I have gone a week or longer without losing a single pound. Each time, the plateau eventually relented and I began to lose weight again. Usually, after getting frustrated with the lack of weight loss, I would undertake to exercise a little more or eat a little less, but I don't think that's what did it; another time I exercised like crazy and ate extra well but lost nothing. All I can suggest is to continue good eating and exercising. Keep at it; your body MUST come around eventually. Slow and steady wins the race.

If this *still* doesn't work, check to make sure you're really only eating as little as you think you are. Calories can sneak up on you. You can consume more than you realize if you don't keep track. I still have to check every once in a while, by counting calories for a few days, to make sure I'm getting only my planned amount, not more.

Some say you should eat more during a plateau, to kick your body out of starvation mode and back into fat-burning mode.

Eating more, exercising less, wishing upon a star … you hear it all. I'm skeptical. It sounds like trying to "trick" your body into shedding fat. I chart my weight every day of the year, and I've *NEVER* noticed my weight go down after I've eaten *MORE* food.

Consider this: years ago, in an effort to synchronize the flow of traffic, New York City put all its traffic lights and pedestrian signals on timers. As part of this, they disconnected the buttons pedestrians pushed to get a "walk" signal. This was all widely publicized, and everybody knew about it. Yet psychologists observed that, years after, people couldn't stop pushing the button, because sometimes the timing would be just right, and the pedestrian would immediately get the "walk" signal. The person couldn't shake the thought that their button-pushing had made the signal change.

I can't help but wonder if it's the same thing here. People who report that their plateaus ended after they decided to eat more might just be reporting the weight loss that their body was already in the process of bringing about. So long as you really are eating and exercising an appropriate amount, your plateau is going to end sooner or later.

I don't understand the mechanics of a plateau. All I know is that if you work with your body to feed it well and give it exercise, it rewards you with health and happiness. Whatever is going on during a plateau, just trust that your body knows what's best, and will come around when it's time.

12 | December: My Last Year of Being Fat

Everything was on track. There was no reason I couldn't finish this by the new year. I had this, right? I was ready to hit my goal and light up like a Christmas tree. Unbeknownst to me, Winter had arrived—and along with its shorter days would come darker times.

Wednesday, Dec 1

7:25 am – Others' interest

I love how people of both genders now look me in the eye when I talk to them. They didn't do that nearly as much when I was fat.

Thursday, Dec 2

8:05 am – Tiny café victory

I'm having breakfast at a lovely little café today. I ordered a gorgeous fresh-baked apricot scone (still a little warm, only moments out of the oven). I put half in a bag for later, being careful to do so before starting to eat, so I wouldn't be tempted to keep going.

It was really yummy and I wanted to eat more. But because I'd already put the other half away, I didn't. Win!

It's a small thing, but I've really been noticing the *small* things can make a *big* difference.

4:10 pm – I'm making a difference?

My weight loss is starting to influence people around me! I have been getting more and more "How did you do it?" questions lately, which of course is really wonderful.

One such wonderful moment was recently at the dentist's

office. The staff behind the desk kept going on and on about my weight loss (they knew me at my heaviest). When I told them some of what I've been doing, one lady, who is quite obese, actually started taking notes while I was talking! After almost ten minutes of chat, she said she was going to start keeping a food journal and go online to find support. So cool!

I was so happy for her. I know she doesn't need to be fat, and I know she must hurt so much inside. I even looked her in the eye and said, "I've been heavy all my life. I know how much it hurts, *right here*," pointing to my heart. I had to say goodbye and get on my way; otherwise, she was going to start crying.

When I started to lose weight, it was for myself. I never thought anyone else would care. Finding that I have been inspiring *others* to lose weight has been just ... I don't have the words to describe it. What an honor.

Saturday, Dec 4

8:20 am – No diet, this

Every time in the past when I've tried a diet, I just *couldn't wait for the diet to end!* But with the changes I've made in my life this year, I'm like, "*End? There is no end!*" I must keep living this way. Soon, it will make me skinny, and once I get there, I'm NOT going back! I plan to stay always vigilant. Because this gives me life. That's why it's a LIFEstyle, not a DIEt.

8:35 am – Cold

The weather got cold a few weeks ago. It's really not helping. Even though I've been getting some pretty awesome exercise lately, I have barely been losing weight at all. I think the problem is the weather, and me not knowing how to respond to it.

In the summer, it was all warm and lovely, and I was happy to be active, and more importantly, I was always in the mood for a cool, refreshing salad or something light.

With colder weather, I'm sluggish and always want to just curl up on my couch at home. When it's time to eat, I find myself looking for something hot and rich. It's hard to find filling hot food that's any good for weight loss, and I have a hard time just chowing down on steamed veggies.

Just another facet of the struggle, I guess.

10:35 am – Trying another long run

Going to try to do 1/4 marathon again. I'm choosing a different route with more hills. It will be a little harder, but the new scenery should help make it more fun.

Did I just say running will be "fun"? That blows my mind.

Sunday, Dec 5

11:00 am – Looks

I'm not bad looking. Wounded heart and messed-up head, will you ever allow me to believe this? – me in front of the mirror this morning

Monday, Dec 6

6:30 pm – Sigh

This is hard.

Tuesday, Dec 7

1:00 pm – War

My stupid flippin' body just hasn't been shedding the pounds like it used to. Barely three pounds in three weeks simply isn't cutting it.

This means war.

Thursday, Dec 9

8:00 am – Finally!

Finally down half a pound after another ludicrous plateau. Half a pound isn't much, but it feels gigantic. It *is* a gigantic relief, for sure.

Six pounds from now, I will set a new record low. That's so close! I can do this.

10:00 pm – Weird times

Lately has been weird. Thinspo hasn't been enough to motivate me. I've been needing to do some soul searching. Been needing to think about how much I want this, about how much I'm willing to give to obtain it.

For months, it became easy. But it stopped being easy weeks ago. I kinda didn't want to have to work so hard for it anymore. I started to take solace in no longer being fat. I considered that maybe "not that fat" might be as far as I make it, instead of making it all the way to skinny.

That thought didn't last long.

I need this. I can't stop now. Getting only to "not that fat" when my heart is set on "skinny" is the same as embracing failure. I've had it with failure. No more. No more giving up. No more thinking I can't do it. I MUST do this.

I'm *going* to do it. Not because it was easy for me. Not because I had a fast metabolism, a personal chef, or some wacky amphetamine prescription. They're going to see me do it because ... because ... I can't even put it into words. Sometimes your heart knows it but your head can't grasp it. This is coming from somewhere deep within, and my heart will never let me rest if I don't do this.

I'm going to do this. I'm going to get skinny.

Friday, Dec 10

1:25 pm – Awesome compliment!

One of the prettiest girls in class said to me today, "You're looking so skinny!"

Considering the source (she would know what it's like!), that's seriously awesome!!!

Saturday, Dec 11

12:20 pm – The heaviness of lightness

I didn't know skinny was so heavy. I'm at the mall again, scratching my head. Am I really seeing this? I'm actually skinnier than average, at least compared to who's here today. I seriously don't know how to handle this fact. My eyes reveal it to me but my heart is too scarred from a life of fatness to allow it to sink in.

I'm so excited to think I am only a handful of pounds away from being legitimately skinny, and maybe even somewhat hot. But it's also scary in a way I simply can't describe. It's uncharted territory. It's like I've almost made it to the end of the rainbow and I'm afraid there'll be no pot of gold.

Who knew that so little weight could be such a big deal?

3:15 pm – Let's go

It's time for another long Saturday run. Seeya several miles from now!

5:10 pm – Did it again!

Just got out of the shower after an EIGHT-MILE run! Another six or seven minutes of running would've allowed me to just eclipse my record, but I was just dead today, as I hadn't planned to run that far, and I failed to bring any water with me. I am so tired I can barely stand, but I'm also deeply satisfied.

Sunday, Dec 12

3:25 pm – 75%

Today I am 3/4 of the way to my goal weight! I have lost 31.5 pounds and have only 10.5 to go! Even cooler than that, I am less than five pounds away from being the lightest I have weighed since … *eighth grade!*

The amazing thing is, I already feel so much better, it feels like I'm *95%* there, not 75%. Something tells me hitting my goal is going to be even better than I hoped. I can't wait to find out.

Monday, Dec 13

10:55 am – Some S's

Something of a *surprise* to me is that *sometimes,* on *some* days, from *some* angles, in *some* lighting . . .

… I'm *somewhat* sexy.

Tuesday, Dec 14

9:00 pm – Slight suckage

I can suck at times. Tonight, I was so happy about a scary final exam being over that I celebrated a little, and wound up consuming about 400 calories more than I should have. Won't be skinnier tomorrow.

Oh well. It will now take a day or two longer to reach my goal. It's not the end of the world, I guess.

Wednesday, Dec 15

7:50 am – Truth and joy

Usually the truth hurts, but I just looked at my driver's license. I actually now weigh *less* than the weight listed (which was, of course, a lie). So sweet!

8:45 am – Just say No

Feeling hungry. Already had breakfast. It's too early for me to need more food. Ignoring.

Thursday, Dec 16

4:10 pm – Others judge by appearances? Say it isn't so!

Today's trip to the mall turned into a fun social science experiment. I wore some clothes which no longer fit me (I had to; it's laundry day). I wore a baggy pair of jeans from when I was bigger and an old top which I really love and can't bear to get rid of, only it's gotten quite huge on me. Nice, name-brand items, but they totally hide my [now somewhat slender] body.

And people were just stupid to me.

Most days lately, I've been wearing new jeans and a fitted top. People pay attention. I even get admiring glances—that sure is new! But today, strangers wouldn't look me in the eye. Not even department store staff would ask if I needed anything.

This was a good lesson. It provided me with another reason to get skinny. People are going to judge by appearances. I can't change that. However, I *can* change *what appearance they're judging.*

Saturday, Dec 18

9:05 am – Most memorable day!

I have to write about my awesome day of feeling beautiful! For some strange reason, yesterday I got more compliments on my looks than I've ever gotten in an entire *week*, from guys and girls alike. Apparently my outfit worked (I was simply wearing a decent-fitting t-shirt and jeans), because I must have had eight or ten people say something at different times!

- I heard the expression "disappearing" from two separate people;
- someone, while complimenting me, motioned with her hands to mimic my sleek shape;
- a chubby guy asked me how I'm doing it because he wants to lose weight; and, best of all,
- a nearby classmate who overheard the above guy ask that question actually piped up with "We were all just talking about how good you're looking lately!" I don't know who "we" is, but it doesn't matter when it's such a lovely compliment!!!

And then it just got better after that! In the evening, a bunch of classmates and I went out to the bar. Before I got there, I changed from my previously-mentioned t-shirt to a fancier fitted top. Well, the mood was *very* celebratory and jovial, and, with a little help from the alcohol, people were definitely letting their hair down and revealing how they really felt about things. Long story short: apparently, I'm actually somewhat hot property! *BLUSH!*

I was getting a *lot* of hugs (not one-armed side hugs, either), I was tickled, I had guys talking to me with their arm around my shoulder, I was playfully *bitten* once(!), and of course I got some petting of my fancy top while hearing how good it looks on me (this sounds kinda sketchy, but these are people I know and trust). The popular pretty girls stood and talked and laughed with me like I was one of them, and the guys seemed to pay equal attention to *me!*

This all sounds highly suspect, at best very shallow of me, and at worst like I would be happy to be molested. Not at all. The whole reason I'm so happy about this is that *for the first time in my life, I felt like a regular person, not a fatso.* Actually, even better than that, I felt legitimately *attractive*.

My head has been spinning ever since. I am walking on a cloud. This is all so new! I think I may have reached the point where I no longer feel ashamed of how I look, no longer assume that others look down on me before they even get to know me, no longer feel like there's anywhere I don't belong because I'm too fat. I think the real me, the sweet, skinny me who was trapped inside that fat body for all those years, has arrived. I couldn't possibly extend a warmer welcome.

11:30 am – Cold rain blues

I really wanted to try a new record-long run today, but it's cold and it's raining off and on. I still may try it, but I'm a little worried I'll get sick.

A minute later

Screw it. Rain or shine, my run starts in ten minutes. Seeya lighter!

1:50 pm – I live to tell the tale

Wound up running 7.5 miles. Not a new record, but still a fine workout. The rain wound up being more of a mist than a downpour, and I burned hundreds of calories. Glad I went!

Sunday, Dec 19

6:15 pm – Zero-loss week

I lost no weight this week. Whatever. My body just screws with me sometimes.

Monday, Dec 20

8:45 am – It's time

What time is it? It's time to get on top of my eating again. My body is not nearly as cooperative as it was when I was heavier. It seems I can lose weight these days only with the strictest of food control. Taking it easy has left me plateauing again.

It seems like I come to this same conclusion every two weeks. Will I learn?

1:40 pm – Mock not, bathroom scale

So sick of the scale mocking me. I'm going for a run.

11:10 pm – Alcohol-enhanced philosophy vs. hypocrisy

- They look at a flower and say, "Oh, look how fragile and delicate! How *pretty!*"
- They look at anything little and say, "How tiny! So *adorable!*"
- They look at anything dainty and finely formed and say, "My, how *beautiful!*"
- They look at something with a sleek, slender, profile and say, "So *elegant!*"
- They look at a girl trying to become tiny, delicate, and slender, and say, "*How horrible! You should be fat and bitter like me!*"

Tuesday, Dec 21

1:15 pm – Ahhhh

Cold run, hot shower. I feel so … cleansed.

Wednesday, Dec 22

7:15 am – Whoa!

Good morning, collarbones!

11:20 am – Hey!

My double chin is completely history! Only when my head is tilted fairly far forward and down does it start to show up, and then only mildly. I really don't mind my face anymore!

3:05 pm – Wow!

Wow, according to my fitness app, I've run 26 miles is the past eleven days. That's a marathon! Now if I can just get that time down to about five hours instead of 264 …

8:45 pm – Déjà vu

Am I *really* no longer fat? At the mall tonight I was struck *again* by how many people are now fatter than I am. I used to always just assume I was the fattest in almost any group of people and leave it at that. Tonight, inside the stores, I'd see myself in a mirror and I'd think *"Not bad,"* but my eyes would home in on the places I saw unwanted bulges, and I'd get sad.

But then I'd go outside and see all the people walking past (I usually try to walk against traffic so I can watch more people) and I was like, *"Wow, I really AM not that bad!"* I'm still more than ten pounds away from feeling like I don't necessarily need to lose weight—yet I am already one of the slimmer ones!

After a lifetime of feeling huge, it is still so hard for me to accept that I'm no longer fat. I wonder if I will always, in my heart, feel fat. Is it so much a part of me that I will never accept it, even if I come to look amazing?

I really am close to looking quite good, if I'm honest with myself. But some part of me deep inside is refusing to let me believe that. Maybe that's a good thing. Maybe I need to always remember the pain of being fat. Because I never want to go back.

Thursday, Dec 23

9:45 am – Results!

OMG finally some results from my hard work! I swear I plateaued for almost two weeks. Often, I *felt* a little skinnier, but the scale was making me *mad!* Well, I finally went to war against my flab; I ran the past three days and ate super well.

But my scale STILL didn't budge … until today. Today, I'm down an entire pound! YES! I am officially *less than ten pounds away* from my goal! I have only single digits to go! I am *going to make it!*

It really pays to follow all that advice you hear about having long-term goals and not giving up.

Friday, Dec 24

10:50 am – Infamous quote verified

It used to be just theoretically true, but now I have first-hand knowledge that, really, nothing tastes as good as thin feels.

3:25 pm – Skinny Christmas to me

I'm so ready for this. I've run six of the past seven days and have eaten smartly. Tomorrow, I'm going to eat as tiny of a Christmas dinner as possible, and the next day I'm going to try to set a new record by running ten miles.

I so badly want skinny. I won't be denied.

Christmas Day

9:10 am – Putting the "Happy" into "Happy Holidays"

Christmas, serendipitously, marks exactly five months of weight loss. Now that Christmas is here, it appears my gift is: *minus 33 pounds*. It seems like a small number and a gigantic number at the same time. It's small because many people have lost much more than that, and because I still have many more pounds to go to until I reach my goal. It's gigantic because losing that weight has completely transformed me from a shameful wreck to a confident smile factory. I am loving my new self so much! It is going to be wonderful when I am finally at the skinny, sexy, healthy weight where I want to be. And I know I'm going to make it there, because this feels less each day like a chore, and more like a calling.

Yes, my weight loss has slowed considerably. Although I lost four pounds in my first *week*, the last four pounds have taken me an entire *month*. I haven't slacked off; it's simply getting harder as I near my ideal weight.

The important thing is, my weight is going down. It would still all be worth it even if I lost only a single pound each month. Because getting thin gives me life.

10:20 am – It's Showtime

Today's the day. I'm mere hours away from Christmas dinner. I am going to rock this so hard. No way will I overdo it and have to suffer such debilitating regret afterward. This is going to be the first Christmas of my life where I don't pig out and stuff myself. And I am going to be so happy about it afterward that I might just start to fly.

OMG I almost accidentally made a joke about pigs flying! So close.

4:50 pm – Yesss!

I did it! Barely more than half a plate of food, more vegetables than anything else, and virtually no mashed potatoes or stuffing. Sweet new record for awesome Christmas eating!

Sunday, Dec 26

9:40 am – Time to break another record

Going for a new record today, as planned. Going to try to run that local ten-mile scenic trail. I need to do this. Because I never thought I could.

2:25 pm – Ten

OMG I did it!—and OMG was it ever hard! The last bit was murder, just murder. Seriously, all those seven-or-eight-mile runs I've been doing lately were child's play compared to this. That 13.1-mile half-marathon I hope to do sometime next year is going to be a serious challenge.

When I finally made it home, I was too weak to stand, or even sit. It seemed like even lying flat on the floor wasn't prone enough of a position to give my body rest. Wow. I have HUGE respect for anyone who has run a half marathon or longer.

Midnight – Late night musings

In the past, I tried so many times to lose weight. Just as many times, I gave up. This time, although I have gotten frustrated with my progress, I'm *not* tempted to quit, because I've seen my life improve so much as I've gotten healthier.

Giving up would make me more miserable than any bumps along the road ever could. In many ways, it would be worse than never starting.

Tuesday, Dec 28

11:15 am – Resisting the Dark Side

In the old days, my favorite thing about the Winter season was all the 20-oz Gingerbread Lattes I would buy. This year, when they appeared on the menu, I promised myself I would have ONLY ONE, for tradition's sake. Yet I still haven't ordered one. Hundreds of calories for only a few seconds of pleasure? I don't think so.

1:00 pm – Another small but wonderful lesson

Although I learned long ago that hunger can often be ignored, I am also starting to realize that being "tired" or "sore" can often be ignored, too!

This morning, it hurt to get out of bed because I was sore from my long run a couple of days ago. I thought, *"Danger! Soreness! Body must rest!"* But then I thought, *"Nah, I'll try a short run anyway, I need to lose this weight."*

Well, to my surprise, my "short" run went longer than I had planned, and soreness was never an issue!

I wonder how many other excuses have been keeping me down when really, all I needed to do was choose success?

7:05 pm – Shallow-ass thought

I've noticed that my butt is finally a butt, not just an ass. Where it used to be just gross and wide and without any shape, it is now somewhat narrow from behind and curvy from the side.

I actually used to seriously think that I didn't have the genetics to have a shapely butt. I didn't need genetics, I just needed to run!

Wednesday, Dec 29

10:45 am – Midnight madness

I awoke at 4:00 am, and couldn't sleep. What to do? That's right, I went for a run! And it was actually amazing.

The night air was perfectly still, a light drizzle had just begun, and there was not a soul in sight. I took it easy, just enjoying the delicious air while listening to the faint sounds of falling rain, my soft and rhythmic breathing, and the gentle pitter-patter of my feet on shiny, damp pavement. It was the most tranquil run of my life. Hours later, I still feel wonderful.

Oh, and I ran for just shy of half an hour without stopping to walk, a new personal best.

Thursday, Dec 30

11:05 pm – Never again fat

One more day 'til the new year. Which means this year was the last fat year of my life.

That's a fact. And a promise.

The new year would bring lower weights, and take me to higher heights, as I kept pressing on. I would begin reaping rewards that exceeded even my already lofty fantasies. However, not all of the lows were weights. You don't just become skinny after living all of your life as a fatso without first experiencing some strangely painful transitions.

Q&A | Motivation and Giving Up

The best thing about today? It comes with a tomorrow.

You desire to create your own success story. One problem: you lack the motivation to make it happen. What can you do?

I reached into my little bag of tricks to pull out the one thing that would inspire you to work hard, pursue your goals, prevail against adversity, and safely negotiate the minefields you must traverse in order to reach your goal. I came up empty-handed. Although the feeling of losing weight and being in control is truly magical, no amount of magic can get you to that place.

You are your own worst enemy. You're an enemy who doesn't fight fair, but uses deception, plays dirty tricks, and sets up ambushes. How can you fight such an enemy? You must simply persevere. You just keep marching forward even after you have taken hit after hit, knowing that you represent a righteous cause, and that you *must* be victorious. In this battle, you represent the good guys, and the only way this story will have a happy ending is if the good guys win.

There's no easy way. You can't do this casually. The cost seems high, but I promise you, it's worth it. In the end, it's a bargain compared to the price of having to endure a life of fat and shame. But the only way to make this happen is to sit down, count the cost, and decide to pay.

Nobody can keep you from succeeding. You know you have what it takes if you *really, truly want this*. You know that the only alternative to taking action is a life of regret. You know that's not the answer. That's not you. That's not the real you.

With the right attitude, and with the work which accompanies that attitude, you can meet the real you. The you who's bound up inside your uncooperative and uncomely body. The beautiful, lovely, happy, skinny you. Even I want to meet that version of you! Why don't you decide, right now, to become the first person to meet the real you?

I know you'll be impressed with who you find.

I lack motivation. Is there any hope for me?

Finding your own motivation is the most important thing, much more so than finding recipes or workouts. Motivation takes an awakening more than anything else. Some honest soul-searching, a real heartfelt examination of yourself, is key to that awakening. You need to ask, "Do I *want* this or do I merely *wish* for this?" It's different.

Some people can eat what they want and not get fat (no, it's not fair—but welcome to life). The rest of us need to choose between enjoying food or enjoying being beautiful, between eating what we want and having the body we want. I don't think there's a way to succeed at this unless you take to heart the [infamous but accurate] frame of mind: "Nothing tastes as good as thin feels."

Yes, there's hope for you. You *can* find your motivation. Sometimes it's hiding, but it's there.

I wish I could be strong, like you.

Me, strong? Not a chance! That's why I was fat all my life! Any strength I now have I gained through my recent perseverance.

Some people have natural strength. Others like us don't. The good news is, emotional strength is no different from physical strength, in that it increases with exercise. A weakling who faithfully goes to the gym will become strong. Likewise, the person who never gives up trying to do this will eventually form the strong habits and sturdy mindset that skinny requires. As will you.

I started out well, but gave up when it seemed like nothing was happening. Advice?

"Nothing was happening"? Don't take this unkindly, but I bet even less is happening now that you've given up. You have two choices: fight or surrender. Fighting doesn't necessarily mean you win every battle, but surrendering always means you lose the entire war.

What do you do in moments when you feel like giving up?

I consider my choices:

1. Go ahead and give up.
2. Keep on running this race.

Choice #1 is automatic failure, weight gain, misery, hating myself, and so on. But I do get to eat whatever I want.

Choice #2 is probably success, happiness, healthiness, contentment. It teaches me to have more consistent self control. It makes others respect me and it helps me to respect myself. It means I will probably live longer and enjoy life more in the process. It means that even if it takes far too long to accomplish my goals, I never have to consider myself a failure.

So yeah. Not such a hard choice after all.

I used to be able to control my eating, but now I don't seem to have any control whatsoever.

This question is a great example of how so much of this battle is in our heads. I know what it's like to "not seem to have any control whatsoever." For some, gaining that control takes a switch of attitude from "I *can* do this" to "I *must* do this." Then again, if you're already saying "I *must* do this," sometimes you need to start saying instead, "I *can*."

I just binged. I feel like such a gigantic, hopeless failure. I want nothing more than to crawl into a corner and puke. How do I pick up the pieces and try again?

You do what you just did and tell someone who understands. You realize you can't undo this, so you quit making matters worse by punishing yourself for it. You think through how you got into this place and you make plans for how to avoid it next time. You forgive yourself. You remind yourself that this is only one day's setback. You look on the bright side and admit that you learned a lesson. You remember that you've got a whole life of success still ahead of you. And you receive this gigantic *hug* from me!

Thanks, but ... I already know all that. Isn't there some more specific advice you can give?

So my "keep on running this race" idea isn't working for you? Here's another way to look at it that may help: don't just keep on running; start *fighting*, too.

If someone tried to assault you (I don't want to use the R word, but that's what I'm thinking of), would you just give up and say, "*Okay, I guess I just deserve this*"? No way! You would fight back!

Likewise with food. Food assaults you. It abuses you. It tries to have its way with you. Don't let it get away with it. Just because you've started a binge doesn't mean you have to let it go all the way with you. *You can say NO to a binge* even after it's already started.

The feeling of power, of freedom, of RELIEF—will be worth the pain of fighting back and tearing yourself away from your attacker.

This all seems so abstract. Do you have a practical tip?

Only this: sit yourself down and figure out that *you want to get healthy more than you want to enjoy full plates of food* at every meal. I mean it. You don't need as much food as you are eating.[13] Our culture has brainwashed you to think that you do. Understand this, and it will become easier to realize you're doing the *right* thing by eating less, *not* an unnatural thing.

I tried eating the way you suggest, but after a week, I had massive cravings. I gave in and ate like crap. Why am I like this? How did you stop this cycle?

Unfortunately, my way of losing weight is *my* way of losing weight, and not the only way. Be careful to find something that works for you. Keep a journal of how you and your body react to different things like eating, exercise, emotions, and situations.

Some suggest a "splurge day" once a week, when you eat whatever foods you want. It helps appease your cravings on a regular basis and it gives you a reward to look forward to after

---

[13] This obviously doesn't apply if you've been starving yourself. If that's true for you, read this as, "You probably don't need as much food as the people around you are eating."

all your hard work. Just try to be careful that your "splurge" doesn't turn into an actual stomach-stretching binge, or it might take you days to recover.

As for me, I never had a "cycle". I just one day decided I was going to embrace hunger, and it instantly started working so well that I never wanted to look back. I had failed in this many times before. I think the important difference this time was *welcoming* the difficulty of the project instead of complaining about how hard it was. If you can adopt this attitude, you will find a strength you never had.

I've actually lost a nice amount of weight, but I fear I'm not going to be able to keep it up. How do I keep on going when my goal seems so far away?

Take a long moment, alone in a quiet place, and visualize what your life will be like if you keep up your good work and get down to your goal weight. Think about how hard it will be to get there … and how lovely it will be to stay there.

Then visualize the opposite. Think of how satisfying it will be to eat whenever you want to … and wake up fatter and fatter each new morning. Think of how life will be after you lost all that weight and were feeling wonderful about it … but then you just gave up and settled for fat.

Then choose your path.

14 | January: A New Year, a New Me (Right?)

A new year about to be filled with new things, among them many new records, had begun. Yay, me … but would I ever reach my goal?

Saturday, Jan 1

8:55 am – Happy(?) Holidays

My holidays were not nearly as happy as I expected them to be. It has been a strange, strange couple of weeks. I decided (and even told people) that I was going to use this time off from school to lose serious weight. I wanted to return to school so thin that classmates, similar to after Thanksgiving, would exclaim, "How did you LOSE weight over Christmas?!?"

I ate well and ran six days a week (my fitness app told me I'd run the equivalent of a marathon every week), but I hit a total weight loss wall. My weight just stopped dropping. I tried to find things to blame myself for so I could change them. But the thing is, I haven't been doing anything wrong. My body has just been uncooperative.

I got even more bummed about it when I heard friends talking about how they'd *lost* weight after days of bad Christmas eating. I thought, "*Obviously my method isn't working. Maybe I need to just relax.*"

So I did. I chilled out.

I haven't done a single shred of exercise for the last couple of days; I merely ate well and tried to have some quality time with friends. This morning, FINALLY, I got some good news from the scale; down half a pound. Unbelievable!

But I would have been okay even if I'd lost no weight at all. Because I need to not obsess. I need my *mind and heart*, not just my body, to be light.

I'm going to stay patient. I'm going to keep on running this race. As long as I finish, I've succeeded. Even the last person to cross the finish line has succeeded.

Sunday, Jan 2

4:05 pm – Thinvisibility

Today, I bumped into a friend I hadn't seen in two months. He actually admitted to not recognizing me when he first saw me!

Tuesday, Jan 4

9:45 pm – Hooray running buddy!

Went for a run today with a (quite fit) friend who visited for the day. I took her on a scenic route through all my favorite spots, and we had the loveliest time. We talked throughout most of our run and just enjoyed one another's company. I seriously didn't even realize how long we were running, it was just so enjoyable.

When we finally got home, I peeked at my GPS-enabled fitness app. Today's was the second longest run of my life! Just short of nine miles. And I could have kept going!

I must do this again. Finding a friend to exercise with is amazing! We ran way farther that we would have run alone, and we had *such* an enjoyable time.

Wednesday, Jan 5

9:30 am – Really gotta try this

I seriously need to get out there and try a half-marathon. That way, when I'm interviewing for a job and they ask about any accomplishments I'm proud of, I can say, "Well, just last summer I weighed almost 170 pounds, and I couldn't run more than ten minutes—but the other day I ran a half marathon."

That ~~would be~~ will be so very cool.

12:45 pm – I don't believe I just did that

I just signed up for a half marathon—and it's in only four

days! *OMG I'm actually going to do this!* Wow. I am both thrilled with my decision and nervous like crazy.

I had originally planned to wait a couple of months to train for it, but I found a nearby race, and the weather is supposed to be decent. I said to myself, *"Screw waiting, I need to *DO* this,"* and I signed up. Just like that. I paid quite a bit of money for the privilege, so I guess there's no backing out. *Gulp*

Best part is, my friend is going to do the race with me! She's never done one before, either. I am SO excited! What a year this is going to be!

Thursday, Jan 6

7:40 am – (Crying)

I am so broken up right now, from the strangest thing. I just finished reading a story in *Runner's World* (first time I've read a running magazine and it didn't seem like it was in a foreign language) about a national championship high-school race. It was a gripping read, incredibly well written. But still, I wasn't prepared for the ending. Background: after running the first mile (of a three-mile race) in 4:46(!), the eventual winner all-out SPRINTED the remaining two miles. Then,

> [The winner] staggered through the chute and collapsed to the grass ... even as the turf cushioned [his] spent body, he couldn't shake the agonies just endured. "I was hurting so bad the last two miles," he said, "I kept going by telling myself, *You only have to hurt another 10 minutes. If you don't keep pushing, you'll regret it the rest of your life.*" [14]

I'm blinking back tears right now. This is so beautiful. It applies so much to the race that each of us is running. It applies to everything in life.

I've been propelling myself with my little saying, "Keep on running this race." It's time to tweak that just a little, as it's no longer adequate. New version: *Keep on running this race—if you don't keep pushing, you'll regret it the rest of your life.*

---

[14] Amby Burfoot, *The Turning Point*, RUNNER'S WORLD. Available at www.runnersworld.com/elite-runners/turning-point

Saturday, Jan 8

8:30 pm – Pre-race jitters

11 hours and 30 minutes until my half marathon. Not that I'm counting. Gosh, I just want to run it right now, I am so pumped! I hope I can get to sleep tonight. Sleep would help.

Sunday, Jan 9

1:35 pm – I did it I did it I did it!

Say hello to the world's newest HALF-MARATHONER! OMG OMG OMG I actually did it! In less than half a year, I went from fat to fit! Holy cow, is this really my life?

I just ran 13.1 miles, shattering my previous record by 2.6 miles (I used to be unable to run 2.6 miles *at all!*). Oh, I am just so elated, it's better than Christmas and my birthday combined! I have been so emotional since my finish. Several times today, I've had to blink back tears as I've thought, *"I'm not just someone who dabbles in running. I'm not even someone who goes for the occasional long run. I am a runner!"* Oh, I feel dizzy, it is so overwhelming.

PRE-RACE: Awoke at 6:15 after a restless night. I was so nervous, wondering, *"Will I be able to do it? Will I fail?"* I met up with B at the race. B is fitter than I am, and a good 15 pounds lighter, but she had never run more than nine miles before (the record she set with me, four days ago). We were both so nervous and excited! B, like me, set no goals other than just finishing.

THE START: When the two of us crossed the line, I turned to B and gave her a high five. *"We've already won, we crossed the starting line!"* I exclaimed. Seriously, just showing up and beginning the race was the hardest part, and now it was behind us. We were already victors.

FIRST QUARTER: I couldn't believe how much FUN we were having! Before we knew it, we'd gone three miles and were having the time of our lives. We were talking, laughing, remarking on other runners, remarking about how happy we were to be doing this together. I've never run an easier three miles in my life. I felt so fresh, it was incredible. We passed the three-mile marker and I said, "Okay, now that we're warmed up, we can start the ten-mile race. Easy!"

HALFWAY: When we passed Mile Seven, B said, "We're over halfway there!" I was like, "Yeah, cool, easy!" but then I thought, *"Crap, that's a nice milestone and all, but we've already been running for about an hour and have almost as far to run."* I started to realize that this wasn't going to be a piece of cake after all.

THREE QUARTERS: At Mile Nine, I was getting seriously tired. I tried comforting myself by remarking, "Guess what? As soon as we pass Mile Ten, that's only 5K left to go! A 5K run isn't that long!" If only it was like that. I was *tired*. Over the next few miles, I had to walk several times. I was getting way burnt out. The worst part was, each time I stopped to walk and regain a little energy, my legs would want to seize up. I needed to walk, but the more I walked, the harder it became for me to resume running. I knew I had to keep running, even taking tiny steps, or I would crash and burn. I told B that once we hit the last mile, I would start running and not stop until we crossed the finish line.

LAST MILE: I expected to feel a surge of energy in the final mile, sensing the closeness of the finish line. Instead, it just got harder. With only half a mile to go, we hit a small uphill section, perhaps only 50 yards of gentle uphill, and I just decided, *"Screw this hill. I need to walk."* But I didn't, because a fraction of a second later, I realized that to do so would be to give up. To admit defeat. To go back on my word. I remembered the race I read about a couple of days ago, and thought *"I need to do this. I need to push myself or I will regret it forever."* I had originally wanted to run the final mile at a fast pace, but I simply had no more to give. I was spent. I jogged slowly and pathetically. But I never stopped.

FINISH LINE: With hundreds of people cheering, we managed to find a little extra strength and pushed hard for the last 200 yards. We crossed the finish line, full speed ahead. At that moment, we won. It took us over two hours. Over two solid hours spent *running*, are you kidding me? It felt like the biggest thing I've ever done. It was one of the happiest moments of my life. I did it. I really did it! I'm no longer a fatso, I'm a *runner*.

Tuesday, Jan 11

8:15 am – Weight loss update

Strangely, I have been stuck on a monumental plateau. I've managed to lose only a little over a pound in the last few weeks.

I'm so perplexed. I don't think I've been eating a ton, and I know I've been exercising a ton.

Whatever.

Wednesday, Jan 12

7:10 pm – Calorie-counting lesson

I counted my caloric intake today. Before, I hadn't been counting for quite some time, as I was just eating small amounts that seemed "right".

Well! Calories never crept up on a person so fast! This leads me to believe I have accidentally been eating more than I thought I was. That definitely helps explain the plateau.

Thursday, Jan 13

8:15 am – Finally, progress

133.4. It may not be as much progress as I had hoped for, but it is still the lowest weight I've hit since starting this weight loss journey.

Limiting my calories yesterday definitely paid off. The best part is: I was never hungry. Oh, I wanted food alright, and had an *appetite*, but I wasn't *hungry*.

I really must have been getting too many calories lately. I wasn't bingeing by any stretch of the imagination, yet it still made me plateau.

6:35 pm – All new clothes!

The last of my old clothes has ceased to fit! Today I am wearing a top which I bought a few years ago, before I ballooned. Recently, I was elated when I had finally lost enough weight to fit back into it. Today I realized it's too big for me!

Next, I realized that *not a single one of my old clothing items fits me anymore.* What a rush!

8:55 pm – Weird gym emotions

Tonight at the gym, I felt both happy and sad. In my fat days, when I would see a fit person at the gym, I felt a combination of *"I will never look like you, I'm so ashamed,"* and *"I hate you, skinny person, because you must be full of yourself."*

Well, tonight was the first time I've gone to a gym in almost a year (if I don't count the workout room at school). Tonight—*so strange*—I noticed a lot of fatter people watching me. Not the usual quick glance and looking away from lack of interest, but eyes would follow me and then they'd dart away when I looked back.

Oh my gosh! I realized that some of these people must see ME as one of the fit ones! I don't think those were *casual* glances, but *admiring* glances. WOW, is this ever a first! For the first time in my life, I was actually NOT one of the out-of-shape people at the gym! It still doesn't seem right after so many years of being chubby. I can hardly believe it.

My elation was quickly tempered, however, by sadness. I felt so *sad* for these people who don't need to be fat. Some of them looked so hopeless. I wanted to shout, *"I wasn't always like this! I'm one of you! I'm proof that you can get into whatever shape you want to be in if you just don't give up."*

So there's my weird heart again. I don't know what to say, I just wanted to get this down. This has been an amazing journey.

Friday, Jan 14

8:20 am – Life like a movie?

In the movie *Mr. Deeds*, the namesake character just went around saying nice things to everybody and making them smile. Oddly, I feel like that's been my life for the past little while.

As I've gotten slender, not only are people generally nice to me all the time, but I've just been so happy so much of the time! Instead of being all moody and dark and down about myself, I have a bounce in my step. People compliment me every day, I thank them and compliment them back … it's just so *lovely!* What a difference from my old life.

6:30 pm – Jeans win

"Those jeans fit you really well." I heard this today at school, regarding new jeans I bought over Christmas Break. That is a serious compliment, if you ask me! Especially because it came from a member of the (ahem) opposite sex! *Blush*

Saturday, Jan 15

5:15 pm – Facebook fail becomes facebook win

After a conspicuous absence, I'm finally back. It has been three years since I last put a picture of myself on facebook. Not coincidentally, three years ago my weight started to balloon. I couldn't bear the thought of revealing to my old friends how gross I'd become.

Today, I'm finally happy to be putting pictures of myself up. I'm already getting positive comments from people who haven't seen me in ages, and they're saying that I look great!

I've lost count of how many ways I never expected to find happiness from losing weight. So many things are now better in my life. To think that I had a *three year* vacation from facebook photos *just because I was ashamed*—and now I don't have to be! It is all so wonderful.

Tuesday, Jan 18

10:00 pm – So . . .

So I wonder what it's going to take to lose these last few pounds. They have definitely not been behaving like the first 35 pounds did. They are tenacious little beasties. I thought I had all this weight loss stuff figured out, but lately, I've been humbled.

No matter. I must press on. The alternative is unthinkable.

Wednesday, Jan 19

10:30 am – Never so happy to be a moron

This is embarrassing. The past few weeks, I've been regular-ly checking myself out in the mirror (as one does when trying to lose weight), and I have been sad that my face hasn't been getting skinnier in one area: in the spot a little below my eyes and in front of the middles of my ears, I have had a little extra "padding" that wouldn't go away. *"Oh, poor me, I have a fat face, look how pudgy it is,"* I thought. WRONG! *Those are cheekbones!* I didn't even know I *had* cheekbones!

I am so stupid! I'm also stupidly *happy!* Wheeee, I have cheekbones! How elegant and attractive is that?!?

Thursday, Jan 20

8:35 am – No way!

IT'S OFFICIAL! I now weigh less than I did when I was a kid! I was under 131 this morning! The last time I weighed this little was when I was *thirteen*—except then, I was several inches shorter, and my body was nowhere near as fully developed.

Unbelievable. This day has been a long time coming. I have been looking forward to it like crazy. Every fraction of a pound I lose from here on will set a NEW RECORD. Every ounce I lose will come with the satisfaction of being able to say, *"I am skinnier now than I have ever been in my life."*

I've come so far that it's starting to get weird to think that I used to be fat. I mean, it was only a matter of months ago, but it feels like such a distant memory. The short-term discomfort of eating less has TOTALLY been worth it, every moment of it!

9:20 pm – Another awesome thing

I've noticed lately that when I tilt my head back, perhaps to look at the ceiling, I can totally feel the skin over my throat stretch taut. I don't know exactly what causes this, but it makes me feel *skinny!*

Friday, Jan 21

7:00 am – Skinny start to my day

I jumped on the scale and I was *exactly* 130lbs! I tried a few more times to see if I could make it read 129.9, but nope, 130 every time. This means that if I eat well today and maybe get a little exercise, tomorrow I should be in the 120s!

Next, after jumping on the scale, I jumped into my jeans. These are the same jeans I bought two months ago, when I had to do all kinds of gymnastics to button them up, and then it took further moves to try to stretch them out before I could go into public with them. Today, they just felt *baggy* on my butt and loose on my hips.

Happy!

4:55 pm – *Human bodies really are weird*

I can't believe that, just a few days ago, I was whining about how my body isn't shedding weight, how these last few pounds are going to be so hard to lose, etcetera. Each day since then, my weight has been dropping like a rock.

None of this makes any sense. But I just keep trying, and my efforts keep paying off. There are no gimmicks in weight loss. It merely takes a good attitude—and a *TON* of patience.

Saturday, Jan 22

9:20 am – *New threshold!*

I made it, YES! 129.4. I can't believe my eyes. That is seriously light!

Sunday, Jan 23

5:25 pm – *Silly new discovery*

Today, I was sitting on a hard wooden chair, which I never usually do. It put pressure on bones I never knew I had, and it was actually rather uncomfortable. I love discovering all these wacky things that skinny people knew all along and deal with every day.

Monday, Jan 24

8:30 pm – *Going with the flow*

So I went for a run first thing this morning because I had a breakfast date planned. Later, I met with a friend for Happy Hour, where I ate a few more nachos than I meant to eat. Result? I ran another 3.3 miles upon returning home. Not because I wanted to, but because it's just what you have to do sometimes to make this work.

Tuesday, Jan 25

10:05 pm – Fascinating change in mindset

Just got in from a run. I ran hard and pushed myself. To my surprise, I actually *enjoyed* how challenging it was. I kind of bowled myself over when I realized that I can find enjoyment from hard exercise.

Oh, how I've changed! I used to run because I *had* to. Now I run to see what I *can* do.

Wednesday, Jan 26

7:20 am – Not fat / New life

I'm not fat. For whatever reason, that's in the forefront of my mind. I want to cry. I can't even describe how heart-wrenchingly beautiful it is to know this. Yes, I still have unwanted flab; still have another jeans size to lose; still have some pounds to go before I hit my Goal Weight. But *I'm not fat.* Even my mirror is complimenting me this morning instead of mocking me. I'm only wearing a t-shirt and jeans today, but I know some eyes are going to follow me. I'm not trying to achieve that effect, it just happens these days. The best part is, I'm not dreaming. I needn't fear waking up and being my old, fat self. That's history.

Saturday, Jan 29

5:40 pm – Motivation evolution

My motivational needs have changed so much.

At first, I needed to look at thinspo all day. Seeing that slender beauty, then tearing myself away from it and seeing myself in front of the mirror ... it killed me and helped me to decide that I didn't want to eat after all.

Later, I just got so happy to be losing weight that it simply became easier to choose to eat well and exercise. More lost weight = more happiness. Simple!

Later still, my mindset changed to "*You've worked so hard and come so far, it would be tragic if you were to be an idiot and undo it.*"

And these days, healthy is just a habit. It feels normal. I get full on a small amount of food, and sitting around inactive actually feels weird.

I guess this is proof of the law of inertia. Once you get rolling, it's hard to stop.

Sunday, Jan 30

2:05 pm – Brrr

Chilly and drizzly today. But today is the only day this week that I have time for a longer run. Guess I'm getting wet.

4:15 pm – So glad I went

I swear, every time I choose to run in the rain, the weather lets up after a while, and I seem to get rewarded for my faithfulness. Today, I ran a path near the ocean, and only about five minutes into the run, the drizzle let up. Within minutes, dazzling rays of sunshine began to pierce the gray, low-hanging rainclouds, breaking them up and revealing a stunning blue sky and blinding white pillows of cloud behind, all which reflected off of and gave color to the darkened sea. To think that I never would've seen any of this had I stayed inside! Instead, I was alone on the trail, and got to keep this glorious moment entirely to myself.

In the end, I ran a total of 7.3 miles and burned something like 700 calories. That's almost my entire day's intake! This all rocks in the most rockingly of rocking ways.

Monday, Jan 31

7:35 pm – New record (small one)

Beat my best 1.75-mile time (15:30) by 15 seconds just now! Considering I was cramping, plus I ran over seven miles yesterday and swam today, I felt pretty good about this. Besides, I *had* to run—the nachos were extra cheesy today.

Cheese aside—and I'll always be cheesy—my life was becoming so different from before that it was hard to recognize the new me, or to remember the old me. Who was I becoming?

Q&A | How Skinny is Skinny Enough & How Quickly Can You Get There?

If your destination is nowhere in particular, you're sure to get there.

In weight loss, there are few truer words than those above. It has also been said, "the odds of hitting your target go up dramatically when you aim at it." Point is, you must set a goal.

The question is, how do you decide on your goal? Setting your goal at "I want to look nice," or, "I'll stop when I'm not fat anymore," or, "I'll stop when I look like the picture of [insert your favorite thinspo here]" is to set disaster as your goal. Even the most beautiful people in the world hate certain aspects of their bodies. Don't think you will fare better. That kind of striving for perfection is what causes people to succumb to debilitating depression, harmful eating disorders, or monstrous amounts of plastic surgery.

There's a funny cartoon going around of a rhinoceros running on a treadmill, sweating like crazy. On the wall, rhino gazing longingly at it for inspiration, is a poster of a glorious, svelte unicorn. Single horn aside, even the world's slenderest rhino will never look like a unicorn.

So it is with humans. Some of us can never look completely like our favorite thinspo, no matter how fit we get. We can look our best, but we have to work with the bodies we've been given. Keep perfection as your dream, but choose reality as your goal.

Why is being skinny so important for you? As long as you're at a healthy weight, whether at the high end or the low end of the curve, you should accept your body.

Before starting this journey, I had been "healthy" before, but never truly slender. People told me I was "not that bad" and that I "didn't need to lose" weight. Thanks, guys, but I was just *tired of being chunky.* I decided it was my turn to learn what being slender is like, and whether it works for me.

When I was fatter, I was obviously unhealthy. I refuse to accept that as being okay. Some say "You don't need to be skinny to be healthy." True. But if it is fine to be at the high end of the curve, and also fine to be at the low end, then it is fine for *me* to choose the low end. Given the choice between loving my body and merely consoling myself with being "not that bad," I choose the former.

I'm X feet and Y inches tall, and weigh Z pounds. How am I doing on a scale of 1 to 10?

I know this sounds odd coming from someone who uses pictures of perfect bodies as motivation, but y*our body is yours, so you should always treat it as if it's a 10.* Keep up good habits, and it will be.

As for your ideal weight, there's no way to pick a solid number. Even if I knew every detail about your body, your ideal weight would still be a *range*, not a number. "Ideal" means healthy and good-looking, right? You can be both of these across a range of different weights.

Also, be careful even of using charts to determine what a healthy weight is. As I've discussed in other places, those charts are for the most average of averagely average people—and that's only on average! A girl who has a large skeletal structure, or well-developed muscularity (either through genetics or exercise), or even a big chest will always feel inadequate using those charts, even if she is skinny. If you happen to be average in every way, then the charts might be meaningful to you. Otherwise, my rule of thumb is: lose as much as you want to lose without it ruining your life, and forget about the numbers as much as possible.

My weight is near the lower limit of "healthy," but I still have quite a bit of noticeable fat. If I lose much more weight, I'll be "underweight". Should I be worried?

Some girls, including many models, are thin but not muscular. They are the first to be labeled "underweight". Yet if the same girls were to hit the gym and develop defined abs and arms, suddenly they'd be considered athletes and role models for healthy living. Isn't it *stupid* that someone with low-fat body composition is considered "athletic" as long as she has abs, but "anorexic" if she has none? The only reason some athletes aren't considered underweight is because their muscle mass pushes them higher up the BMI charts (well, and also because they look beautiful and it's hard for others to fault anything about their bodies) when, in fact, they are extremely thin.

To be truly "underweight" means that a person has too little fat to correctly perform certain bodily health functions, NOT merely that the person weighs too few pounds for a certain height. You can be healthy and skinny if you eat right and do at least a little bit of exercise. If you, like me, are genetically pre-disposed to have low muscle mass, a healthy weight might still nudge you into the "underweight" category. If that's the case, there's probably little need to panic. If you're not missing any periods, you're not fainting or frequently cold, your blood chemical levels are good,[15] and your hair isn't falling out, you're likely healthy.[16]

As an aside, you might also be what they call "skinnyfat". This describes people who aren't technically overweight but also are soft and flabby. Such people often never exercise, and that's the root of the condition. When skinnyfat people start working out, they lose the fat—but they don't enter the "underweight" zone, because they don't actually lose weight. The exercise causes them to gain a little bit of attractive muscle where there was once fat.

In conclusion, as always: eat little, and exercise some. And remember to stay beautiful on the inside, without letting a little bit of fat control how you view yourself.

If I eat tiny amounts and run every day, can I lose ten pounds in just a few weeks?

It depends. If you're already at a fairly low weight, it's harder to lose weight than if you're quite heavy. Still, I used to lose two or three pounds almost every week, so you can probably lose that weight in that time, if you are serious about it.

---

[15] Learning what these levels are is part of a good physical exam. It might cost a little more, but I highly recommend asking your doctor to do some "blood work" on you. It can be a great way to see how your body is behaving "behind the scenes".
[16] Unless your doctor tells you otherwise … listen to your doctor!

However, as always, I recommend a long-term outlook over a short-term goal. Remember: *if you lose ANYTHING, you're a winner!* Don't get stuck thinking it MUST be a certain amount by a certain time. Instead, develop good habits that will last a lifetime.

My goal is much more serious. I'm starting at a new school in six months. I want to lose 70 pounds by then. Is that possible?

Possible? In theory, yes. Advisable? Only if you want to become a very unhappy person. I know you're frustrated, but setting up such a lofty (and probably unhealthy) goal may drive you crazy. Worse, if you don't succeed, you will hate yourself for it—and perhaps even unravel and go back to your old ways.

Here's a better idea: change your lifestyle, starting today. Make it a permanent change. Let your first day of school be wonderful no matter what you weigh. Later, enjoy basking in the praise of your classmates as they watch you continuing to get healthier. This way, they won't just dismiss you when they first meet you ("Oh, there's just another skinny girl"). Instead, they will come to admire you.

I know what I'm talking about. This is exactly what happened to me.

Most people say I'm already quite skinny, but ... I'm not happy. I have no confidence and I'm always hard on myself. If I lose weight, maybe I'll be happier.

Sometimes we don't see things, especially things about ourselves, all that clearly. If you lose weight and still feel the same way, I would urge you to talk to an actual therapeutic counselor. I used to think they were creepy, but I later learned that an experienced therapist can be amazingly helpful. It's rarely like you see depicted where you lie on a couch and talk about your childhood while some disconnected old man scribbles notes about you. Instead, often, you find yourself with someone who cares, who is the best listener you've ever met, who knows how to ask just the right questions to help you figure it all out.

Being skinny isn't enough to make you or me happy. It only makes one part of our lives more bearable. Please keep that in mind, or you'll be quite disappointed when you get there.

16 | February: More Tortoise than Hare

My progress had seriously slowed. I couldn't figure out why. I tried to keep things positive, but the lack of success was quickly growing old. I could redouble my efforts ... or I could let up and just savor what I'd accomplished.

Wednesday, Feb 2

8:30 am – My skinny new life

It's been a little over six months. So far I've lost 38 pounds, or 9/10 of the weight I set out to lose. Inside, I feel like I've already arrived. I have no doubt that I will soon be at my perfect, most lovely weight. My life has changed so drastically, I pretty much can't describe it. I am going to try anyway.

Everything. That's what's better in my life now. *Everything.* I can't think of a single thing that isn't somehow easier, more joyful, more hopeful, or otherwise improved. In every facet of my life I am happier and more capable. Being fat crippled me in countless ways. Getting thin has allowed me to throw away my crutches and run. It has been nothing short of miraculous.

When fat, I walked this Earth a prisoner. My fat was a straitjacket, my appetite a ball and chain. By way of analogy, victims of severe strokes are said to be completely mentally alert, but they are unable to respond with their bodies; they are trapped, silently, inside. That is how I felt when I was fat. Inside, I was this cool, fun, attractive person, but the real me was covered—*smothered*—by my fat. I was so lonely. It's like I came to attend a party but I was locked out, pounding on the window, looking in at everybody having fun, and not being noticed.

Now that I'm [fairly] skinny, it's like I have busted out of my straitjacket and burst onto the scene. The Real Me is finally, brilliantly, on display for all the world to see. I feel resplendent. It's not just in my head, either: people these days, friends and strangers alike, give me the red carpet treatment wherever I go. People look me in the eye. No—change that. People *gaze* into my eyes. People used to dismiss me in a heartbeat, but now it seems I have everybody's attention.

I cringe writing this, thinking I must surely sound full of myself. I protest to the contrary: I am completely bewildered by it all. This is all in such sharp contrast to my former life that it probably seems to me like a greater difference than it really is. But I cannot deny that it is happening to me every day. I have confidence because I'm no longer ashamed. I have joy because I feel like I'm victorious. I smile because I can't help it. People smile back, they listen to me, they compliment me, they flirt with me, and, most importantly, they seem to respect me. On the inside, I'm the same person, only stronger and happier. On the outside, however, I am an entirely new person—in many ways, unrecognizably so. I'm fond of saying "Thin Gives Life." Well, it does.

Then there's my body. I actually enjoy examining it. I can spend long moments caressing my ribs, hipbones, collarbones, shoulders, cheekbones … the list goes on like Anatomy class. I awake in the morning and feel the flatness of my tummy; I stretch, and feel my taut skin gliding over my frame. I have greater flexibility and can reach places on my body I formerly never could. I open my closet to an entirely new wardrobe, because not a single old item fits anymore. I slip into my jeans instead of stuffing myself into them. I put my head and arms into a sweater and the rest just falls into place instead of needing to be pulled down. Out in public, I'm no longer in the habit of blousing my top away from my body, even when a breeze is pressing the cloth against me. I walk past shops and rejoice when the glass is angled toward me so I can check out my reflection without actually having to turn my head and make it obvious. For the first time in my life, I am happy with how I look.

Finally, on the inside. I could write pages on this. Suffice it to say that not only have I become happy with how I look, I am now happy with who I am. Some people say that getting in shape gives them "energy". For me, it's more than just energy, it's also hope. And it's peace. To borrow from my poem *skinny*, this experience has put a song on my lips and a spring in my step. I have vanquished the foe I never imagined I could defeat and I have become the person I never dreamt I could be.

7:30 pm – Stress relief

Was feeling all pent up and stressed out from errands and homework. Went for a run. Now everything is okay. I love how that works.

Thursday, Feb 3

11:20 am – Fail

Teacher brought donuts to class. This genius ate a large one. Guess I'm skipping lunch now.

Sunday, Feb 6

9:05 am – Operation Finish Line starts NOW

For two weeks, I have been slacking off on my eating. Unsurprisingly, in that time I've lost 0.000 pounds, give or take .000 pounds.

I am too close to my goal to let myself stagnate. I am going to try to eat *super well* and thus lose four pounds in the next two weeks. If I am successful, I will finally hit 125.

This is so going to be worth it if I can pull it off!

5:30 pm – Another role reversal

Went for a run this afternoon with my incredibly sweet and slender friend L. We used to jog together when I was fat and I would be wheezing, begging to walk, and she never complained, even though I was majorly slowing her down.

Well, yesterday was the first time we've run together in a couple of months, and this time *she* was the one needing to stop and walk. I could have left her in my dust, I was barely even breathing heavily! She even confessed that now things are the opposite of how they used to be. I didn't respond other than to tell her that she was always 100% wonderful to me before, and I'll always be grateful for how much she supported me.

L is a beautiful girl. I've admired her—and envied her—for years. Now I'm a better runner than she is, and almost as skinny. Sometimes I really love my life these days.

9:25 pm – OFL Day One report

First day of Operation Finish Line went pretty well. I got in a medium length run and ate really well, including salad for dinner.

Looking forward to waking up skinnier tomorrow. I hope, anyway. I should. Right?

Tuesday, Feb 8

10:45 am – On course for success

Two days of Operation Finish Line have yielded a 3/4-pound loss. Yes! If I can keep this up for a whole two weeks without messing up, it should work.

I SO want this. I can endure two weeks of suffering if it means I cross the finish line. Oh yeah.

7:20 pm – Skinny people have it easy?

Saw a cute comic. A somewhat heavy girl was snacking on chips and offered some to a slender girl standing nearby. Slender girl declined, saying she was on a diet. Heavy girl gasped and did a double take, staring at this perfect example of beauty, wondering how she could possibly need to diet.

This totally hits the nail on the head. I used to think those girls were always skinny naturally, not because they had to work on it. Just today at the café, I told the girl behind the counter that I wasn't going to buy the cookie she offered because I needed to lose weight. She was incredulous. I felt awkward. Awkward but triumphant.

Wednesday, Feb 9

7:35 am – Morning glory

Good morning, scale! Thanks for lowering that number by another half a pound!

6:20 pm – Who is this person?

I'm discovering what I look like. And I'm just stunned. *I never knew that I never knew.* This is so deep. A lifetime of being fat left me completely ignorant about one of the most fundamental things about me.

I just got out of the shower and I was looking at myself in the mirror, and I thought, "*Wow, my face looks really nice!*" And then it hit me: *before* now, *I never knew what I looked like.* I mean, obviously I don't look unrecognizable, but until lately (and especially today), I never knew what *the real contours of my face* looked like. Today I realized I can see the spot on my face where my (newly discovered) cheekbones become my cheeks, then where my cheeks become my jaw, and where my jaw line merges into my chin. Before, my face was just round-ish. Then it got more oval. Then it got kinda blocky oval. And now it has very little fat left on it, and since I took the time to examine it more closely, I finally learned, for the first time, how I look.

This is so weird. The changes in me really have been profound and unexpected.

Friday, Feb 11

12:15 pm – Should've known

After three awesome days of weight loss in Operation Finish Line, as I so gallantly called it, I stopped losing weight—and then today my weight even crept up. Should've called it Operation Fail. Because now I'm no longer even in the mood to try.

This is why I don't "diet". I did better when I just tried to eat better EVERY day, instead of trying to "sprint" for a short time. Setting goals of "I must lose *x* pounds by *y* date" is setting up for failure. I wanted to shed four pounds in two weeks. Yet if I had kept going and lost only three, I would have felt like a failure—when in fact I'd have lost three pounds, which is awesome!

I'm choosing to be content with whatever weight I lose, no matter how much it is and no matter how long it takes.

Sunday, Feb 13

10:05 am – Ugh

Craving that large strawberry chocolate truffle across the room. Going to try to make tea instead.

Today, I'm 127.8 pounds. So, so close!

7:50 pm – Revelation

This morning, the weather was unusually warm, so I wore shorts. Standing in line at the café behind a somewhat heavy girl, also in shorts, I noticed her calves were a little round and unshapely, and I was like, "*Ugh. She has the same unflattering calves I do.*"

Then I glanced down at my calves and I was like "*OMG! I have slender legs, not fat legs! And I can see toned calf muscles!*"

My mind still hasn't caught up with my body. I wonder if I will ever stop feeling fat. I know I'm not fat, but I still can't believe it.

Thursday, Feb 17

6:25 pm – C'mon already

For almost a week, I've been giving in where I used to triumph, enough to completely halt my weight loss and gain most of a pound. Example: I ate about 250 calories of chocolate yesterday. I *never* do that! So weird. I hope it's just a phase I'm going through. I'll get over this. It's not worth it.

Midnight – Moodiness gone

Was really moody earlier, upset about gaining weight. Went for a run; problems gone. Few crummy moods can't be solved by a good workout.

Saturday, Feb 19

2:20 pm – This is doable

I didn't police my eating this week—and I gained two pounds. I feel so stupid. But it's only a week. No reason to hate myself. I'm still going to do this.

Wednesday, Feb 23

11:00 pm – Tough times make tough people?

After being all down about last week's two-pound gain, I finally got a grip. The weight is now gone, and it feels great to be on track again. This stuff just happens, I guess. I suppose this struggle will never cease to be a struggle.

The most important thing I've learned is to think long term. For almost a week, I felt like a failure. But if I don't think of this in days or weeks but as something I'm going to do for life, I'm no longer a failure. I merely hit a bump in the road, like everyone does from time to time. I'll become a failure only if I give up.

Thursday, Feb 24

5:25 pm – Best skinny moment yet

Strangely, my favorite "skinny moment" to date happened while I was wearing the most clothing. Today, I interviewed for a job. I showed up in my brand new tailored outfit, and I just felt so professional. More than that, having lost so much weight, I felt *gorgeous*. I was just *brimming with confidence*. It was AWESOME. I looked good, I felt good. I radiated confidence and competence. Thin Gives Life!

Monday, Feb 28

10:35 pm – Glad this month is over

Now that February is about to end, I've officially lost … 1.5 pounds the entire month. That makes me almost sick, it's so crappy compared to my first six months. But what are my options? Give up and embrace the fat, or keep on running this race? There's no contest.

Winter. It wasn't pretty, but it didn't last forever. Like Rome wasn't built in a day, a person can't just decide to instantly become skinny overnight. A person can, however, promise themselves each morning, "Tonight I am going to bed healthier than I awoke." That was the plan, anyway.

Q&A | When Others Get You Down

What prevents you from obtaining your goal? What insurmountable obstacle stands in your way (and it has to be insurmountable)?
You can't answer that, can you?

People who mean well and people who think evil toward you; both can frustrate you and make you miserable by resisting your efforts to lose weight. Even those who don't care one way or the other unwittingly set traps for you by tempting you with food you really don't need. Fending off these sources of distraction can be tough. It requires forethought and determination.

Anyone who's lost weight and started looking good has discovered this resistance. You're not yet skinny, and you're obviously FAR from looking anorexic, so *what is these people's problem???* Chances are, it's either (1) they're genuinely concerned and think you'll take this too far, resulting in harm to you; or (2) they envy you and wish *they* were the ones losing weight and looking awesome. Either way, go easy on them.

If they're in the first group, and are merely concerned, be glad that someone cares. They've all heard ED horror stories and don't want you to become one. They've also heard that anything less than 1200 calories per day is "starving yourself". They mean well. If these aren't people you can simply ignore, you need to either set them straight about nutrition, or convince them that you aren't going to fall into an ED, or both. Just be honest with them, and also with yourself. Remember: often-times, the people around us can see us more clearly than we see ourselves. Don't ignore them if they are being reasonable.

The second group of naysayers, the enviers, will likely dwarf the first by a huge ratio. Humans are simply envious by nature. Admit it: even you envy others who are better-looking. We just don't like seeing others better off than we are. Factor in those crazy emotions wrapped up in our ideas of personal attractiveness, and we REALLY don't like to see others better off. Yes, envy is wrong, but it's also hard to combat, even in yourself. Don't let it get you down, just recognize it as a fact of life.

Whichever the case, when the inevitable negativity comes, *be gracious*. When you do, you become the role model. When you don't, you cause others to ramp up their efforts to resist you, to gossip about you, and even to resent you.

In the beginning, everybody was so supportive when I said I wanted to lose weight. These days, however, I keep hearing that I'm just going to gain it all back, or that we'll all be fat once we have kids, or that it runs in the family, etc. Why all the discouragement instead of being happy for me?

The negativity is the strangest thing. It teaches you about people. People love to praise you about your weight loss—that is, until you start looking better than they do. I'm just glad I never stopped when people told me to stop. May you also teach everyone a lesson by continuing with your success—and showing them how wrong they are.

My friends are really starting to nag me about my eating. I've been losing weight the healthy way, but they try to guilt-trip me about my eating "too little," or they try to dissuade me from exercising. How should I deal with this?

I've noticed a pattern. Friends skinnier than me either tell me not to worry or else they congratulate me for wanting to lose more. Friends fatter than me (of both sexes) tell me not to lose any more. The worst offenders are the friends who used to be skinnier than me, but have watched me get skinnier than them. One in particular began to constantly call me "anorexic" and taunt me for eating "rabbit food".

In every case, however, once I did lose more weight, EVERYBODY congratulated me and raved about how great I look. Even the one who felt the need to call me anorexic eventually admitted that I inspired her to lose weight.

[Time out. It's confession time: not long ago, this same girl, who used to be visibly overweight, recently shared, online, a picture of herself in a bikini. She looked somewhat decent. I'm ashamed to admit that my first reaction was not to think how happy I was for her. Instead, I found myself disappointed that I was no longer so much skinnier than she was. Even after all this transformation of heart and mind I've gone through, I still succumbed to that feeling of not wanting others to be as successful as me. This is all further proof that negativity from others is unavoidable—and neither is it something you should care about in the least.]

So, in conclusion, how do you deal with your friends? Don't take their comments personally, because they obviously don't know what they're talking about. Ignore them if you can. If you need them off your back, tell them that you're trying to get *healthier*, not that you're trying to get *skinnier*. Who can have a problem with that?

My coworkers have noticed the healthy changes I've made to my eating, and they've suddenly started offering me sweets and treating me to lunch, which they never previously did. I swear, it's like they're hoping for me to fail.

Other people *do* want you to fail sometimes, even if they don't realize it. However, don't rule out the possibility that it's just coincidence, and that you are feeling especially vulnerable in this time.

As for me, once I started losing weight, it felt *so good* being on the path to skinny that I wasn't willing to let *anybody* get in my way. People would tell me. "You're not fat, you don't need to lose weight!" I'm sure many of them were just trying to make me feel good about myself the way I was. I appreciate that they were trying to be nice, but it's a good thing I didn't listen to them.

In your case, just picture your wonderful future skinny self, then dig your heels in. Thank your coworkers profusely, but insist that you have eaten enough already. They will let off, or they won't. Either way, the only way you will triumph is by not giving in, so don't. Your coworkers aren't the ones who have to look in your mirror every morning.

What do you do about meals with others? They all eat so much more than I am trying to eat.

Eating near others is one of the hardest things. You see them stuffing their faces and you want to do the same. They also tease you about how little you're eating. If they won't accept "I need to lose weight" as a reason, try, "I'm being careful to fill up with only good foods, and to limit other foods." Even if you don't say it out loud, say it to yourself.

Just keep up the good work and, one day, rather than taunting, "C'mon, have some more!" they will instead gush, "No wonder you're so tiny! I wish I had your self-control."

I lost a lot of weight a few years ago, but plateaued at "almost there." My husband swears he loves my body as is, and that I needn't lose any more. How do you explain to someone close to you that you need to lose weight when they disagree?

I just pinch my fat and show them, saying, "Thank you for your support. I want to lose a little more weight, and *it's something I need to do for me.* If ever you see me starting to get *too* skinny, please speak up then, and I'll listen to you."

Until people begin to become legitimately worried about your health and they sincerely ask you to put on weight, I don't think there's much need to "accept" having a fatter body than you want. If in doubt, ask your doctor if your goal is healthy. That should steer you straight, and it should help to settle the argument back home.

Family dinners are ruining my weight loss. I really don't want to eat as much as everyone else does, but it feels like I must. What do I do?

First, do everything you can to make sure your portions are as small as you would like them to be. If that leaves your plate with too much empty space, add some vegetables or salad (stuff you should be eating lots of in the first place).

Next, start off eating slowly from the very beginning (and talking a lot, if the setting permits), so you can make your portion last longer. If you don't, you will soon be sitting there motionless, watching everyone else merrily chomping away while your plate is empty. Not only is this a strong temptation to add more to your plate, it invites all kind of "Eat, eat!" comments. You don't need that kind of pressure.

Chances are, you're still going to face questioning on why

you aren't eating more. Say as sweetly and sincerely as you can, "I'm trying to teach myself self-control." This sounds much more mature, and much less alarming, than does "I want to be skinny."

I have a different family dinner problem. I go all day eating awesomely, but when I arrive home, my mom will have spent a long time making really delicious but fattening food, and I just have to eat it. Problem is, that single meal winds up being so high in calories, it completely undoes my whole day's eating.

Gosh, this is a tough one. Sometimes making the right choice really hurts. What has given me strength in times like this is remembering that the pain of rejecting food is far more bearable than the pain of rejecting myself. I find joy from being able to say No because it means I'm on my way to skinny, but I find shame from feeling full and knowing I didn't need to eat all that.

When you're down to a healthy weight, you can enjoy a greater amount of Mom's cooking. Meanwhile, when you are traveling home, fearing to sit down to supper, you should at the very least *plan out in advance* how much you're going to eat. Picture yourself saying "No, thank you" to second and third helpings. Picture serving yourself half as much as you've been eating, then slowly savoring each bite for twice as long. Picture yourself going to bed with a big grin on your face and a faint grumble in your tummy. Contemplate the joy you will have each morning when you step on the scale to see a lower number, and when you look in the mirror to see a cute face that's not all puffy. It really is better than the extra food. But it takes a conscious choice.

My family won't cease harping on me for "eating too little". How can I convince them I'm not anorexic, but am merely ready to cease being chubby?

The family who jumps on you is quite the foe. I doubt they can be easily convinced. If my above advice isn't working, I'm guessing the only thing that would help is if you do some research and show them that X number of calories can be fine for you as you're losing weight. Consider keeping a food journal to show that you are getting that many calories and that you're going about it in a health-conscious way. Be warned, however: if you're shooting for, say, fewer than 1000 calories per day (like I do when I'm losing weight), it's going to be a challenge to convince anyone that it's healthy. Funny thing is, I've never been healthier. So ironic.

18 | March: "Springing" Back

A new season was just around the corner. Surely the arrival of Spring would mark my rebound from such a disappointing Winter?

Tuesday, Mar 1

2:20 pm – New feature

I'm enjoying the veins in my hands. Not because they're particularly attractive, but because for so long they were obscured by fat. Hi veins!

Wednesday, Mar 2

8:15 am – Liking my scale again

The scale finally cooperated a little! It has been SOOOO long since the number has actually moved down. Today, I'm half a pound lower than ever. I've got only 2.2 pounds 'til I hit 125—but WOW are these last few pounds ever tenacious!

Saturday, Mar 5

7:35 am – Hooray for even numbers

I've officially lost *40 pounds* today! It feels so good to hit such a big number. It really sounds like progress when I realize that 40 pounds is like a third of what I currently weigh!

I know others have lost this much weight in less than half the time it took me to lose it, and it makes me feel like I suck at weight loss. Maybe I do. I don't care, because no matter how long it took me, those 40 pounds are permanently gone. Gone, baby, gone!

Sunday, Mar 6

8:10 am – Happy accidents

I actually bump into objects with my hipbones now and then. It makes me so happy.

11:05 am – Sweet compliment

A friend told me that she overheard someone we both know commenting that they'd never seen a transformation in a person like they've seen in *my* weight loss!

Gah!!! How cool is that?

Thursday, Mar 10

5:45 pm – Unashamed

Sometimes, you've got a secret you're hiding, something you're ashamed of, but which you need to tell somebody. When you finally do confess, it's such a relief. That was me today at the beach.

When I got to the beach (being careful to sit as far away from anybody else as possible), then stripped to my bathing suit, I suddenly felt a strange flood of relief. Instead of feeling naked and just somehow *wrong*, like I always felt at the beach before, today I felt *triumphant*. I felt like I had finally overcome a huge hurdle, like finally confessing something I had been hiding. In a way, for all those years, I *was* hiding. I was hiding my fat under as much clothing as possible.

Today, it almost felt like I had *repented* from my wrongs. It was a profoundly liberating moment. Just me, the ocean, the sun on my skin, and, for the first time in my life, not even caring if anybody saw me. Because I'm no longer ashamed of my body. A little embarrassed, yes, but not ashamed.

Friday, Mar 11

9:40 pm – Ashamed

It's so stupid that I'm not yet at my goal weight. I've not been feeling the same motivation that I used to, as I'm no longer shamefully fat. It's gotten much easier to splurge instead of maintaining that strict control that made me lose all that weight.

I don't yet know what it's going to take to propel me to victory. I know I have it in me, but it's like I am fighting against myself. I want to be skinny, but I want to celebrate how skinny I've gotten ... by eating.

Monday, Mar 14

8:35 am – What?!?

OMG what if my scale is telling the truth? No, it's too good to be true. But still ... !

My scale reported 125.3 this morning. *That's almost two pounds less* than yesterday morning! I know it's not real, because I went for a long run yesterday, and I'm certain it's because I haven't replenished all the water I lost, but STILL: *I FEEL and LOOK wonderfully skinny today.* I am so happy, I might just start floating away!

Friday, Mar 18

12:55 pm – Why, hello there, neck!

Just got in from a run. Odd thing: while running, I reached up to scratch my neck for a second, and instead of feeling flab and double chin, I felt tight skin.

It still never ceases to amaze me: I've gotten somewhat skinny! Lord, it's so awesome.

Sunday, Mar 27

1:15 pm – Eight months plus

It's been over eight months since I started eating well—and I don't miss my old ways at all. The idea that this is a "lifestyle" is *true*. It CAN be done! And I'm GOING to do it.

9:30 pm – Goal reassessment

I'm almost there. So I need to start thinking about what I will change when I reach my goal. I guess I'll just keep weighing myself daily, trying to exercise, trying to be smart about what I eat. I've come to realize that I will never be able to pound back the junk food like I used to, and I'm okay with that. The rewards of skinniness are worth it to not allow that vice in my life anymore.

Speaking of goals, I'm changing mine. I set 125 as my goal way back when, not knowing how I would look or feel at 125 (I've never been that light!). I recently decided that I need to set my final "ultimate" goal weight at 120. I'm looking decent in clothes, but I still have some unsightly flabbiness that I would like to be rid of. I don't seek unrealistic perfection, only to be as good as I can be without being underweight. Once I'm there, I need only stay smart about things.

Tuesday, Mar 29

7:45 am – Hotness: gift or reward?

Early this morning, just a few minutes after dark o'clock, I saw a cute, skinny girl out for a run. She looked perfect, and I thought, "*No fair! Why can't I look like that?*"

I immediately caught myself. There's nothing unfair about it. *She* was the one out running when most people were still in bed.

And you know what? I *can* look like that.

Thursday, Mar 31

8:00 am – Movie plot life

Just like in a movie storyline, our heroine is within moments of reaching her goal and saving the world (or in this case, she's less than a pound away from reaching her Goal Weight), yet from out of nowhere comes a horrible sequence of events threatening to lead to her imminent demise. Egad!

This weekend, I have a series of events and parties to attend, all with tons of food and some with limitless free drinks. And I have been looking forward to it for months. Gah! Old me would be stoked, but new me is freaked. I am SO close to my goal! What do I do?

I'm just going to try to tell myself all weekend: "You are going to remember this time in one of two ways. It can be either a short-lived memory of good food and good times, or a long-term memory of victory in the face of overwhelming odds. The former will fade into the memories of every other such occasion; the latter will shine forever in your heart and mind."

I'm going to try so hard, I'm really going to try. I don't want to blow this. I want this movie to have a happy ending.

Will our heroine prevail and save the world, or will she succumb to the hostile conditions threatening her very existence? Find out next time, in the April episode of Eat To Live or Die Eating!

19 | April: Is THIS the Moment?

The ending of my "movie" was just ... whatever. I "won" in the sense that I didn't go crazy and stuff myself, but I consumed enough that it certainly wasn't a Hollywood ending. Back to work.

Monday, Apr 4

1:50 pm – Fat head

Although I acknowledge that I've come a long way, I am still super conscious of the little fat I have left. My self confidence is almost non-existent, because I spent my entire life, until now, fat. That pain doesn't just go away. I guess it's a healing process.

3:15 pm – I sound so schizophrenic at times

OMG my [hot] classmate called me a "twig"! What a sweet compliment!

Tuesday, Apr 5

4:20 pm – Lesson in averting failure

I went for a run. I thought I'd do four miles. Problem is, I had no fuel in my tank. I got very tired very quickly. I wanted to turn around early and make it a short run.

But I didn't. I decided to make my run *longer*. This way, I reasoned, I could walk more often, yet still get in the full four miles of actual running. I wound up doing 4.9 miles, and wound up walking only about 0.3 of those miles! So cool! By asserting a better attitude, I actually had a *better* workout than I had originally planned.

This is so different from my old way of thinking! In the

past, I chose the easy way simply because I disliked the hard way. Now, I choose the hard way because the easy way feels like giving up.

5:55 pm – *Winning by cheating!*

I just weighed myself. I know it doesn't count because I had lost a lot of water weight, but I was 124.5, half a pound under my Goal Weight!

We will see what I look like in the morning. Let's just say I'm pretty excited.

Wednesday Apr 6

8:05 am – *Soooooo close I can taste it*

Still not officially at 125 this morning, but if I'm really, really, really good today, and as long as my body cooperates, I think I might hit my goal tomorrow!

Thursday, Apr 7

7:35 am – *Aw, c'mon already!*

Still not at my goal. WTH? I guess it was water weight I lost, after all. No matter, I'm going to DO this.

Friday, Apr 8

9:10 am – *FML*

Still not 125? Is this some kind of joke? Whatever. I've lasted this long. You can't outlast my resolve, body!

Saturday, Apr 9

8:40 am – *No comment*

The following is all I have to say about today's visit with the scale: "_____."

Sunday, Apr 10

8:05 am – V-Day

Oh. My. Gosh.
124.9.
Wow.
Wow again!
Although I've always tried to stay positive, and tried to act as if nothing was going to stop me, truth be told, I seriously never knew for sure if I would actually be able to lose any real weight. I'd tried and failed so many times before. I was worried I would keep up my flawless record of failing at every attempt to use self control.

I guess it wasn't so impossible after all.

I would normally write on and on about this, but this is too big of a moment, and I'm still trying to figure out how I feel. I have been ready for this day for so long. Now that it's here, I don't even know what to think. I just feel very … quiet. I'm not jumping up and down with glee, but I'm not choking up, either. I guess I would summarize it by saying I'm just so, so … *content*. And I'm just so *ready* to get out there and introduce the Real Me to the world.

Monday, Apr 11

3:40 pm – This is real

Today it's starting to sink in. I really am at a great weight. I really am skinnier than most. I really am not bad-looking. I really did do it. I really don't think I will ever be fat again. I really might cry.

Tuesday, Apr 12

11:30 am – More deep thoughts

I've been contemplating a lot lately. Something I've realized is that it actually, somehow deep inside … *validates me as a person* to not be fat anymore.

It's not that skinny is all there is to life. Far from it. But fat can certainly keep you from experiencing life.

This is the real me, not the almost me nor the camouflaged me nor the wounded me. This is the whole me. The me I was designed to be.

Monday, Apr 18

3:15 pm – NSV!

Had another Non-Scale Victory! Today's was in a league of its own. For a long time, I couldn't cross my legs properly. Like, the ladylike way, where one knee goes above the other knee instead of with an ankle resting on top of the opposite knee. I used to have too much thigh fat to be able to comfortably cross my legs that way. For a long time, I never even tried.

But, moments ago, my legs were crossed the other way (the "wrong" way), and I was wearing nylon hiking pants, which were somewhat slippery, and my leg sorta just slid on down until it flopped over the other, knee on top of knee. This is so silly. But so meaningful.

9:10 pm – How I plan to keep it all off

Many people have asked me a variant of the question, "Have you thought about how you're going to maintain your weight once you're satisfied you've lost enough?"

It's like this: since I was never "afraid" to eat food like some girls are, it's actually a pretty easy change. I'll just relax my standards a little and *voilà*, I'm eating as much as I should be eating.

I am certainly NOT going back to my old ways. For a long time now, I've known this was going to have to be a lifestyle change. And, well, my life *has* changed, and it really doesn't feel like I'm on a diet. I've learned a new way to live, a way marked by self-control and a sense of victory, accomplishment, and worth.

Tuesday, Apr 19

9:15 pm – The camera lies?

I video-chatted for the first time tonight! It was so weird seeing my face as portrayed by webcam: I looked skinny! I'm used to seeing myself in the mirror, which is always the same lighting, always knowing what to expect, not really seeing myself as others do.

During the video chat, I could see my image while talking. I couldn't believe it; I finally saw what others see when looking at me, and I was amazed to realize that I really don't look fat anymore! The camera doesn't lie, right?

Happy sigh

The healing process is underway. Tonight was a real victory.

Sunday, Apr 24

5:00 pm – It's still all in the attitude

I must confess something. I gained over half a pound since hitting my goal weight. And it has been there for a few days, so it's not just a fluke. Today, I think I figured out why.

I've gotten complacent. Yes, I have developed pretty good eating and exercise habits, and I have NOT AT ALL returned to my old ways, but lately I've been permitting myself to eat noticeably more than I used to. And I'm apparently paying the price.

I still want to lose another three or five more pounds. And I guess I took it for granted that I would keep losing weight, because that's what I've done virtually every week for the past eight months. I thought that since I'm still being fairly mindful of what I eat, it should be easy. Not so. If I keep slacking off, the weight is NOT going to come off. I need to quit "celebrating" and get back to my "*Let's DO this!*" frame of mind.

I figured a slightly milder effort would mean a slightly slower weight loss—but it has actually meant NO weight loss. I need to remember what I've already learned. I need to embrace the difficulty, not shrink from it. I need to *do this* for me, and not just *hope it happens* to me.

In the beginning, I assumed that reaching my goal would bring my story to a close. However, many of my most profound changes were yet to come. You don't just begin life anew without noticing some pretty bewildering things.

Q&A | Finding Motivation When You're Almost There (and Beyond)

You can be happy to eat what you want or happy that you lost the weight. Choose your happy.

The Boston Marathon features one of the most notorious uphill sections in all of running, the legendary "Heartbreak Hill". It's barely a third of a mile long, rising only 88 feet in elevation. But because it shows up later than the 20-mile mark of the race, when runners are already spent and exhausted, it's a killer. It's said that once you crest Heartbreak, even though more than five miles remain, you've essentially made it to the finish line.

Likewise is the latter part of your weight-loss journey. You started out well, and you lost so much weight. Life is now *really* great and you're in many ways a new person. You've made it so far, and have only a short distance to go until you reach the finish. Then you hit this hill. And it shouldn't be very hard, but it is. You know that the way to overcome this obstacle is to charge hard at it. But suddenly it seems like so much work, and you don't know if you have the strength do it.

Worse, the novelty has worn off. The excitement and challenge of your new weight-loss routine has become mundane and burdensome. The euphoria of losing weight when you never thought you could do it has been diluted by all the praise you're receiving now that you look amazing. The urgency of shedding weight has waned. It's no longer like you're being chased by a bear, but you are now just irritated by a yapping poodle. Your thoughts are no longer "*I'll do whatever it takes— just get me out of this fat body!*" but "*I sure would love it if I was a little bit thinner.*" Your current weight isn't bad. You could stop now and be happy … or could you?

Perhaps you could. There's no actual *need* for anyone to be all-the-way skinny. You can stop at "healthy" and live an amazing life. Frankly, if you're the kind of person who obsesses about her weight, you probably *should* stop at healthy, for your own sanity and happiness.

However, that may not be what you really crave deep down inside. If you need instead to finally know what it's like to be at your *best* weight, the weight where you can comfortably look at yourself and say "*I don't need to lose a single pound,*" know that new challenges will arise as you close in on your goal. The target will have moved. Even though you've already experienced much success, you will need to find new ways to reach inside and find the strength to rise to the occasion, to meet these challenges, and to surmount your own Heartbreak Hill.

I've been behaving really well for months, and have lost most of the weight I want to lose. But for the past month, I've barely lost anything. It's now so hard to eat well. How do I get over this?

My weight also came off much more slowly as time went on. I don't know all the reasons for this. Some of it was physiological (the less overweight you are, the less quickly you tend to lose weight), but some of it was because I lost my extreme NEED to get skinny. I wasn't truly FAT anymore, only a little too heavy.

So what did I do when I faced this similar situation? I realized I must choose between:

1. giving up and resigning myself to remaining "almost skinny"; or
2. pushing hard until the end.

Only the second option would reward me with joy and satisfaction rather than with guilt and embarrassment.

I know that the race course gave you an unwelcome surprise by having an uphill section close to the finish line. But come on—it's the *finish line!* And it's *right there!* You can do this. It will feel like it is too hard and like it is taking too long, but once you're there, you will wonder where all the time went. And you will have *won.*

I lost a serious amount of weight, but lately, I've been slacking off. I was fine for a while, but suddenly my weight shot up and I feel like crap. What do I do? I can no longer seem to convince myself to avoid indulging in bad foods.

Forgive me, but, simply put, eating more of such food will make you unhappier, while eating less of them will make you happier. I wish I could put it in a way that would magically make sense to you, but I can't. I know how hard it is to take this to heart, I really know. But seriously, you must sit yourself down and decide between continuing to do what you're now doing (and continuing to gain weight), or [you fill in the blank].

I'm only a handful of pounds away from reaching my goal. I'm afraid that once I'm there, I'm going to gain the weight all back, because this all seems too good to be true. Any tips for the final stretch?

Remember that skinny must be something you do for life. You can't go back to your old ways. Once you reach your goal, you're not "done," you just shift gears a little and prepare for long-term success.

When I hit my goal, I got a little lazy—and put on a little weight. I had a *really* hard time shaking off those excess pounds, because I had gotten into the habit of enjoying my meals a little too much. I swear, it was more difficult to make small changes then than it was to make the large changes I made in the beginning. I'm afraid you will always have to be careful—as must I, to this day.

What do I do when I actually hit my Ultimate Goal Weight?

After you're done with all the dancing, yelling, and crying, you just enjoy it for a while! You're *skinny! You! NOT* someone else, *NOT* that girl who's always been skinny, but *YOU!* Lavish in the *sweetness* of your victory. Take some time out to think about *what just happened.* Don't get down on yourself by obsessing right away about how you're going to work super hard to make sure you never get fat again. Just enjoy the new you and give thanks that you've arrived.

Then, of course, you *will* actually need to implement a maintenance strategy. And you will need to do it soon, to avoid the demoralizing blow that weight gain would give you after such sweet victory. How do you do this?

Maintaining weight is actually quite different from losing weight. When you're losing weight, you have this bright light at the end of the tunnel, your *Ultimate Goal Weight*. Your goal motivates you and helps you succeed. Once you meet your goal, however, you MUST take measures to preserve your success, because you will no longer have the power of The Goal to keep you going. You're like a ship arriving at a distant harbor after an arduous journey. You can have survived a thousand perils, but unless you put your anchor down, you're going to drift back out to sea.

In weight loss terms, I recommend you set a new goal, or install an alarm system, or both.

By "new goal," I mean a fitness goal, not a weight goal. If you're at a healthy and happy weight, you definitely don't want to ruin things by continuing to get skinnier. Rather, you can get faster, stronger, more toned, more flexible, better at a sport, or any combination of the above. Find which of these most appeals to you, and set an appropriate fitness-based, rather than a weight-based, goal (but please do remember that gaining muscle makes your scale report a bigger number, so don't freak out when you're heavier but not fatter). After you meet this goal, set another.

I'm actually a bad example of this. Before I ran my half-marathon, I was running six to ten miles most of the times I went out. That's because 13.1 miles was my goal. In the entire *year* following the half, however, I ran greater than six miles so few times I can actually count it with my fingers. Probably on one hand. That's what happens when you lack a goal. What did I need? I needed to set my goal for either (a) a lower time in another half marathon, or (b) *any* time in a full marathon. Although I have yet to complete either feat,[17] setting this goal inspired me and propelled me to resume longer, more focused runs.

Next, let's talk about installing an "alarm system". What do I mean by this? You need to regularly check yourself to make sure you're not accidentally creeping up in weight. I seriously recommend that every person keeps a daily weight chart. I keep mine right in my bathroom, and update it every morning. If I notice the line angling upward, it has a doubly effective impact on me. First, I think *"Crap! I gained weight again!"* Next, I look at the graph where the numbers were lower in the past, and I contemplate, *"I was there just a little while ago. That felt awesome. I*

---

[17] But watch out for the next edition of this book!

must get back, pronto."

You can use other means to measure how you're doing. Actual tape measuring of your waist, hips, arms, and so on can alert you to a bulge that would otherwise go unnoticed. Regularly trying on your favorite item of skinny-sized clothing also reveals much (and remember: if it's jeans, it doesn't count unless freshly washed!).

My favorite advice, however, is to take a ton of pictures of yourself when you're at your goal. Pictures with friends, pictures in the mirror, pictures of you smiling when you're at your loveliest weight. Pictures of you when you feel just awesome in your new body. When you put on a few pounds, you will look at those pictures and say to yourself, "I had that! I wasn't born with it, I had to work for it. It was really hard getting there. But I did it—and I can do it again."

That is the ultimate thinspo.

21 | Summer of Skinny

It was time to experience life as a skinny person, and there was no better time to do so than Summer. But there were important questions that I was unqualified to answer; questions like what does skinny life even look like, how do you share it with others, and how do you avoid screwing it up?

Friday, May 6

1:40 pm – So sweet

Five people in the last two days have complimented me on how skinny I've gotten! It never gets old.

11:25 pm – What goal do I set?

I feel a little aimless. I met my Goal Weight, but I'm not yet at my Ultimate Goal Weight. I actually don't know what that weight is, because I don't know what weight it will take to make me happy.

I know I can lose the weight, but something's missing. Is it complacency? Am I burnt out from school? Am I as skinny as I will ever be? Where do I go from here?

Sunday, May 8

7:40 pm – Interesting turn

My old friend who used to call me "anorexic" just told me that she can't fit into her old slacks anymore, and she wants to take me up on my offer to share with her how to lose the weight once and for all.

It's amazing how my weight loss, which was always just a personal goal, is affecting other people. I feel like I've really accomplished something worthwhile. It's not just about me.

Wednesday, May 11

12:20 pm – Mind blown

Wow, even people who knew me when I was fat don't think of me as fat! Today, some friends at school saw my student ID photo (taken last summer) and just gasped, saying, "I don't even recognize the person in this picture!"

That just blew my mind, because I figured that since they met me when I was fat, they would always think of me as fat. How wonderful that they don't! This is a small detail, but it's huge.

Thursday, May 26

11:00 am – Travel = Good

I am now on a huge summer travel excursion—and I am getting skinnier! With the combination of being too busy to get bored ("bored" is when I am most tempted to eat) and also because food is too expensive where I am, I have been eating way less since arriving—and I can totally feel the difference! I don't have access to a scale, but my tummy feels noticeably flatter and I think my reflection in the mirror is smaller, hooray!

Travelling is awesome. I'm not stuck in a rut like I was back home, where I would come home at the end of the day and open the refrigerator. Plus, I'm exploring on foot, getting in lots of walking and even a few runs. I love it!

I was afraid to go on this trip without a scale, fearing that I would plump up without realizing I was gaining weight. But if I can keep up my weight loss attitude even while on the road, I should be able to make serious progress!

Friday, May 27

7:55 am – I'm not fat even by European standards???

I am in *Europe* and I *don't* feel fat—even though almost everybody here is skinny!

I never pictured myself being able to say this. I mean, it's one thing to be skinny compared to others in America, but when I'm on the train in Europe and I see plenty of beautiful girls who have bigger thighs and butt than I do … GOSH it feels wonderful! It really does pay to watch what you eat.

Sunday, May 29

Noon – Strange moment of reckoning

In less than a year, I've transformed from "self-loathingly fat with hope for the future" to "joyfully thin with gratitude for the present." I'm sad to report, however, that some things are still just crap.

I'm visiting an awesome place filled with beautiful people. For weeks, I had planned for and envisioned myself coming out here and experiencing the coolest nightlife. I had been fantasizing about how glorious it would be, like some kind of a Cinderella moment.

Well, it's Sunday night. And I never went out this weekend. Even after all my planning, I just found myself choking on fear and lacking self-confidence. All my fantasies aside, I couldn't shake my self-doubts. That voice inside my head kept saying *"You're fat and ugly. You've always been fat and ugly. If you try to be friendly and cool, others will see through it and taunt, 'Who the hell are you?' and you will feel like the biggest loser."*

It's so weird. I really think I've become decent-looking. I've had people express to me (not just my friends, either) that they think I'm attractive. But I just haven't been able to take it to heart. After a lifetime of being an outsider to the cool crowd, and of always being rejected and feeling sorry for myself, I still don't know how to have any confidence in the real world. In my fantasy world, sure, but in the real world, I'm still the old, scared little me inside.

I don't know what to do. This weight loss stuff can be … foreign.

Monday, Jun 6

12:20 pm – Done

I finally fulfilled my dream. I went out to a trendy club. I didn't focus on how ugly / lame / stupid I felt. Instead, I just had an amazing time. I felt awesome. I even attracted some attention!

I still don't care much for nightclubs. Not my scene. But I did do some growing up and some figuring myself out. It was amazing.

Oh, and … I'm pretty sure I was among the good-looking ones in the club. Not all puffed up about it, but I did get hit on pretty seriously, by someone rather hot, who could easily have chosen anyone else.

Monday, Jun 20

11:30 am – Road Trip? Try Run Trip!

Amazing! I was visiting a glorious new city for only a short time, not enough time to see everything. So I decided to see the city by JOGGING over substantially the whole downtown area! OMG I never enjoyed exercise so much! The run was I-don't-know-how-many miles (perhaps ten?) long. It took me well over two hours, but, to be fair, I was stopping frequently to take pictures.

All I did was take a map, stick it in my pocket, and go. I ran down every street that looked interesting, past every landmark that seemed important. Whenever the street I was on started to bore me, I tried a different one. Since I was having so much fun, I was able to run *much* farther than I was used to running. The freshness of the scenery just propelled me on and on. It was amazing! I was so absorbed by the beauty, I barely noticed I was getting exercise.

It was serious fun blasting past all the waddling tourists and even most of the locals. I felt alive, I felt beautiful, I felt gleeful after having had a bad day yesterday of feeling too small in a too-big world. Now, afterwards, my body feels absolutely dead—but I am buoyed by joy from this accomplishment.

Plus, I burned easily more than a thousand calories, so it's time to reward myself with [a small amount of] food and drink—and an excursion to see if there are any charming locals to be found!

Friday, Jul 1

5:45 pm – Slimmer still?

I haven't weighed myself in a month and a half, so I don't

really know what my weight is doing, but I'm pretty sure I've lost a little more. Even if I haven't, I feel slimmer, and my formerly loose skin seems to be tightening up.

Some other recent non-scale victories I've been savoring:

- Lying in bed each morning and running my hands over my flat tummy, rippled ribs, and pokey hipbones really is still the most *amazing* thing.
- Walking around and feeling my shorts kinda *swish* around my butt and hips (instead of *squeezing* them tightly) makes me feel light and free.
- On the train the other day, reaching up to retrieve my bag from the overhead shelf, I noticed my reflection in the window. My shirt had risen to show a little bit of my tummy—and there was *no hint of muffin top!* Also, my jeans were riding a little low on my hips, and you could see a tiny sliver of underwear peeking out! Can't lie ... I felt sexy.
- Speaking of, the jeans I refer to are my "reward jeans" which I bought many pounds ago, hoping that someday I might fit into them. I figured they were the smallest size I could ever possibly fit into ... but I think, pretty soon, I'm going to need to go down a size.

I am so happy with my new body! Food could never satisfy me as much as being skinny is satisfying me.

Wednesday, July 5

8:45 pm – Lightness

I had such a good eating day today. It just makes my heart feel *buoyant!*

Sunday, Jul 10

10:30 am – Screw-up

Guess who screwed up?

Yeah, so a couple of days ago, I was having an awesome eating day, and I was so proud of myself. I even ate a salad for lunch when I had wanted a large hot sandwich instead. I was out with a couple of friends in the evening. They wanted to get dinner. I said I would be happy to join them, but that I really didn't need to eat any more that day. I said I would help pay, and maybe have a bite off of each of their plates.

At the restaurant, my friends each ordered a big entrée, then said, "Why don't you go in with us on the appetizer platter?" I felt bad thinking I would be just sitting there watching them eat, so I agreed. When the platter arrived, I caved and ate all kinds of crap that I didn't need. Deep-fried crap. Some vegetables, too, but mostly crap. I didn't binge, but I sure didn't stop at "just a bite off of each of their plates."

I felt like the failiest of failures. I went from feeling super triumphant from my great day of eating to feeling super filled with angst and regret.

I went for a late night run a few hours later, just to make me feel like I wasn't totally out of control. The running was jostling the contents of my stomach and I kept tasting reminders of my stupid, unnecessary meal.

So. Why even mention this? Just to remind myself that crap happens sometimes. It will always be a struggle, I suppose.

Wednesday, Jul 13

1:30 pm – Beach lessons in thinspo

I've been at many beaches this summer, beaches in different countries and on different continents. The thing that has surprised me most is that *there is hardly any thinspo at the beach.* Girls all over the place jiggle a little when they walk, and they spread out when they lie down. Yet for the most part they look like normal, healthy people.

This reminds me that *the thinspo world is not the real world.* It's good to use thinspo for inspiration to get healthier, for sure, but not to use it as a standard, to think of oneself as a failure if one doesn't look like the pictures—because hardly anybody does.

Sunday, Jul 17

Midnight – Anniversary

I'm restless, as I ponder that I'm only a few days away from the anniversary of my weight loss journey's beginning. Fifty-one weeks ago today, after days of reading people's stories, and seeing how hard it was for them, yet how successful they were, I decided it was going to be my turn. Both of these things came true: it was hard—and it was my turn.

It has taken me months since reaching my Goal Weight to adjust to not feeling like my body is my enemy anymore, to not feel *fat* anymore. Not until this week did I realize that I finally, legitimately don't feel fat. Until now, there has *NEVER* been a time in my *LIFE* that I haven't felt fat, or haven't identified deep inside as a fatso. Today, I still would like to lose a little weight, but really, doesn't almost everybody? I may be a little embarrassed by some bulges here and there, but I'm not *fat*. In fact, I almost can't believe I used to be fat, because the new skinny me seems so natural, so real, so … *me*.

Apparently, nobody else sees me as fat, either. When in the past strangers would have given me indifferent greetings, today people seem almost universally warm when I meet them. I'm sure some of this is just that they are reflecting my newfound attitude when I approach: because I'm no longer ashamed of myself, I no longer project my unhappiness and timidity to others. My poise is more confident, too, because I don't feel like I need to hide behind myself. I'm even ceasing to make comments to others about my being soft or flabby, because every time I do, people give me the strangest looks, and I feel like I'm almost offending them by thusly referring to myself. Frankly, I think I get it. In reality, I've actually become thin and fit compared to many people. For me to say "I need to lose weight" must make others uncomfortably self-conscious. This is such a strange twist from all my years of feeling inadequate every time I compared myself to other people. It has taken a long time to sink in. I've still got a way to go, I know, but in the meantime, it just rocks my world. I want to cry when I think about it. I'm not fat. Did you hear that? *I'm not fat!!!*

How not fat am I? Though I'm not yet completely satisfied with it, I do love my new body. Almost every time I pass a mirror, I find myself surprised at the good looking reflection smirking back at me. I half expect it to wink. I can't believe that I actually have a fairly attractive face, a face that I never fully knew until now because it was hidden all those years under a layer of fat. Now and then when I see my reflection, I actually notice those subtle lines where you can see shadows on my neck, throat, and collarbones when the light is hitting me just right. Same with my legs where the muscles of my calves ripple a little when I walk. Heck, even my knees are looking better than ever! I am constantly finding new things about myself that I like, new reasons to be thankful for how much I've changed.

I'm also way less self-conscious about my body when I'm around others. The beach is still a fairly foreign place to me, but certain things that used to make me cringe no longer do. When someone puts their arm around me for a picture, and their hand rests on the side of my waist, it's no big deal. When I sit down in shorts, I don't try to rearrange my thighs to look like they're not spreading out too much—because they aren't! Even if someone gives me a shoulder rub, which I used to hate because I knew they could feel my fat shifting around, I relax and even think silently, *"Check out those bones, baby!"*

My body is also so much healthier and more capable than it ever was. Running isn't even hard for me anymore, and I no longer feel out of place amongst others working out. I can also stretch more easily, reaching places I always thought impossible. Heck, I'm even exploring new places when I do stretch: who knew I could actually feel my shoulder blades when simply scratching my back? And when did I get vertebrae? Best of all, are those *really* back dimples I feel??? Yes, dear, they are, they really are. They're not much, but they're there, and they're *yours!*

Finally, there's the subject of food. Food used to be a savage predator lying in wait to ambush me. I feared it almost as much as I loved it and, like an abused woman in a bad relationship, I felt powerless to resist it. Today, food no longer frightens me. In fact, it's really no big deal. I just eat what I need (and sometimes what I crave, but only a little bit), and I've stopped seeking to soothe my soul by forking food into my face. Rather than pining, *"It's so goooood! I want morrrrrrrre!,"* I instead think, *"That was delicious. I'm happy I had some, but I'll be seriously UNhappy if I keep going,"* and that's it. I don't count calories anymore, I merely eat small meals. I'm never hungry, because it just feels normal and natural and *right*.

Furthermore, if ever I do eat an amount close to what used to be a normal-sized meal for me, it actually makes me uncomfortably full, and it's hard to digest. I sometimes actually stagger at amazement seeing what my friends can put away (eek, what I used to be able to cram into *me!*), because I'm sure my stomach could never fit that much food today. I can't say that I never eat more than I should, but I can say that, for the most part, I'm now the one in control. It's not even something I think about, it's merely part of who I've become. Eating less is now something I naturally desire, because it just feels so good to be *free*.

So here I am, a year after seeing my first thinspo picture. Even though a year sounds like a long way away when you're looking at it as a future event, this entire past year seems like but a moment. The pain and hardships of losing weight seem brief and insignificant in my memory, whereas my joys and victories from losing that weight feel huge and permanent. It really wasn't a sacrifice, *it was a bargain.* It wasn't deprivation, it was *liberation.*

How is gold refined? It's put through the fire and melted down to remove all the impurities. It's an intense process, but it's worth it because the result is precious. Similarly, not one— *not one!*—of the changes I made in my life over the past year was comfortable or natural to me at first. But I had faith that if I kept it up, the rewards would exceed the regrets. I had no idea how right I would be. All I wanted was to stop hating my body, yet I progressed far beyond that. I found an even greater treasure than I could have expected. I really have found new life.

Thursday, Jul 28

12:35 pm – I found a scale!

I've not wanted to weigh myself while traveling, but the place where I stayed last night had a scale and I was just too curious.

Unless the scale is way off, I've lost three pounds since May! Considering that I've been doing far too much eating out, including eating too many carbs, this is awesome! The good portion control habits I've taught myself are paying off, even though I can't often find the healthful foods I like to buy back home.

Happy!

Saturday, Jul 30

9:20 am – Wow, lost more than I thought I did!

Yikes, I officially lost over four pounds since May! This morning, I'm a hair under 121! Considering my original Goal Weight was 125, this is amazing!

New jeans are most definitely in order.

Sunday, Jul 31

6:40 pm – On attraction

My summer has been so amazing in so many ways. One of the most amazing things, however, is that I have realized something incredibly deep, even though it's incredibly shallow. I know this sounds really stupid at first, but: I'm a little bit *sexy*.

I said it sounds stupid! I really am SO not full of myself! This thought actually *bewilders* me so much! I lived all my life wondering why others were good-looking but I was somewhere between homely and hideous. As a child, I got picked on for being chubby. As a teenager, I never went to dances, and I completely skipped going to prom (as if I could even have found a date). Why make myself feel worse by feeling ugly and suffering rejection? Inside, I always knew I was unattractive.

Now, everything is different.

This summer, I met hundreds of people in over a dozen countries. None of them knew my past, they only saw the current version of me. And they were *attracted* to me. I got hit on time and time again. Since I'm not used to that happening, even my friends had to point out sometimes when someone was flirting with me, and my first instinct was always to say, "No, you're making that up!" because I really didn't believe anyone would be into me. But after it kept happening, I started to figure it out and even came to believe it.

In my past, the kinds of guys who liked me were usually the ones who stood little chance themselves. I'm usually friendly with everybody, and many so-so guys (and that's being slightly generous) liked me probably just because I was kind to them. Lately, however, things have been very different. It finally clicked when I realized that the homely guys (I know that sounds mean, but I can't think of a better word) had stopped hitting on me. I think it's because, in their minds, I'm *out of their league.* These days, to my frequent surprise, it's actually *cute* guys who flirt with me! The ones I always thought were out of *my* league! This is so bizarre, in some ways it makes my head spin. Is this really happening? Am I really now fending off advances that I previously wouldn't even have dreamed of? Wow, yes, I am.

So. Why go on about this, especially when I'm not into random hookups? Because it is evidence of an amazing change. This ugly duckling has become a swan. I never knew I had it in me. I thought all my life I was doomed to be an also-ran. I didn't even think that I had any good genes, figuring that when I lost weight, I would just be a skinnier and happier version of my old, ugly self. *And I was completely okay with that!* Yet it turns out that there was someone more beautiful hiding beneath my fat than I had realized. This realization has given me a monumental increase in confidence, which makes everything else in life better, too.

It's true that it's what's inside that counts. But if you can package that beautiful being on the inside with healthy beauty on the outside, you become even more resplendent. You radiate. You bless others with your presence, and you reap personal rewards you never thought possible. Is it really important in the big scheme of things? Of course not. But will you regret a minute of it? Never. Because thin gives life.

22 | Surf Lessons: Year Two and Beyond

My year of weight loss was like learning to surf: it felt impossible at first; and once I tried, I fell down countless times; but before long came the exhilaration of riding wave after wave of awesomeness. Problem is, like I said in the beginning of this book, "The only direction you can successfully coast … is downhill." Likewise, if you try to ride the same wave forever, you'll wash up.

THE BLESSING OF THIN

After my one year anniversary and all the bliss it brought, and after my preposterous little note on sexiness, things … actually kept getting better.

Saturday, Aug 6 – Strangers are stranger

Wow, this is amazing: even people I don't know are now complimenting me on my weight loss! I had two neighbors today mention that I've lost so much weight and I'm looking great. I don't even know who they are! One lady asked me how I did it. I told her, in general terms, and she said my story inspires her so much, she now has hope that she can do it. What an honor!

Imagine if I had listened to all the people who told me many pounds ago that I shouldn't lose any more weight but I was fine the way I was.

Uh, NO.

My perspective on life and the world changed for the better, too:

Monday, Sep 26 – I'm thin. Now what?

My life is so much better now that I'm no longer fat. So, so much better! But in many ways, life still sucks. In some ways, it's even harder than it was before.

Getting thin makes life *better*, but it doesn't make life *good*. It means some things are *easier*, yet still almost nothing is *easy*. It means *better-looking people* like you, but not *better people*. And it doesn't make you a better person.

Is it worth it? Of course. Is it The Answer? No, and it can never be. Getting thin is a good goal. But it's not *THE* goal.

Exercise got easier.

Sunday, Oct 23 – I killed the 5K!

It's been a year since my last 5K, and I knew I could run faster this year, but I had no idea I would be more than SEVEN MINUTES faster!!! OMG that's so huge it's like the difference between jogging it and walking it. Or in my case, the difference between jogging it (last year) and running it (this year).

I *LOVE* weight loss!

Compliments got awesomer.

Saturday, Nov 19 – New title

I got called a "beanpole" today!!!

Weight loss became a piece of cake.

Monday, Dec 19 – Portion control WORKS

Someone I just met said to me, out of the

blue, "So what do you do? You must run or bike or something."

WHAAATTTT?!? Is that not an *awesome* compliment?

Funny thing is, I've been running only about once a week for the past three months, because my schedule has been too draining to leave me energy or willpower for exercise. Yet I didn't gain weight! Actually, just this past week I have been extra careful about my eating and I've already lost a pound and a half.

THIS IS POSSIBLE!

I started congratulating myself on how I had this all figured out. Easy! Permanent change! Not a diet, a lifestyle! And so on.

Thursday, Dec 29 – New skinny habits

I don't count calories these days, so I actually don't know what my intake has been of late. My weight has been stable for four months, so I'm doing alright, whatever I'm doing.

I know one thing for certain, however: I still eat way less than I did back in my fat days. I really have changed my lifestyle. I have developed what is probably an optimal intake for myself. It's less than my friends and most other people eat—BUT I also now weigh less than most of my friends and other people do.

I remember the night I wrote the above note. I had been checking myself out in a full-length mirror before jumping into the shower. I was the lightest weight I'd ever been (120.5) and seriously slender. I stood sideways to the mirror and stared at my stomach, which was completely flat. Not a single bulge anywhere. When you've never known anything in your life other than fat, you don't forget a moment like this. The image is seared into my brain.

But there was one big problem. You've heard of a blessing in disguise. I was about to meet a curse in disguise.

THE CURSE OF THIN

I no longer needed to lose weight. I'd hit my goal and surpassed it. I was happy with how I looked. You'd think this would be wonderful, but it was actually hard to stay positive about eating well, because the excitement and mystery of weight loss had vanished.

Then came a new year, and with it an extremely busy and stressful schedule, plus certain crappy things going on in my life that drained me of energy and happiness. I got mildly depressed. Well, not so much depressed as just *over it* and a little pissed off at the world. I so badly needed a break, but I was too busy to take one. I craved a way to comfort myself. I chose badly: I started eating and drinking my way to happiness.

Truth be told, I wasn't actually eating all that much. A year and a half of losing and maintaining my weight didn't just go up in smoke. I'd developed really good eating habits, and they felt natural to me. I wasn't about to abandon them.

But I *did* start having a drink most evenings after I got home. When I was so stressed out and unhappy, it was a quick fix, a way to brighten my mood. But the problem with alcohol is more than just with the calories it contains. It also lowers inhibitions and the ability to control impulses. And it really tripped me up. After a drink or two, I would get the munchies. With my self-control diminished, I found it really easy to give in. I'd eat well all day, then succumb to that ancient evil, the evening snack—or, often, snacks.

Saturday, Mar 24 – Failure

I'm a failure. I gained six pounds in the last ten weeks. That puts me back over my goal weight and makes me feel like crap. I feel fat, I feel unattractive, I feel like a loser, my new skinny clothes now fit tightly ... the list goes on.

Right now, life is hard. Food and drink are a comfort. But they're also the enemy. They're not a solution, they're a problem.

I'm neither anorexic nor bulimic. I'm just human. I like to eat. It provides instant comfort. It provides pleasure. It satisfies.

Only it doesn't. At least not for the long term.

In some ways, I'm a weight loss success story. But I must still face the facts: weight loss is seriously difficult. It requires determination. It requires patience. I read today that the Latin root of the word "patience" means "suffering". Yes, weight loss requires suffering. But, like everything worth having … it is worth whatever it takes to get there. It is worth the suffering. It is worth the patience. Patience will be rewarded.

I'm going to go get out there and experience the rewards of my patience.

Full of resolve and ready to lose the extra flab, I went out into the world and … did nothing. My plans never materialized, because, shortly after, I received some distressing news, and it left me scrambling to keep my wits together. I was so stressed out and unhappy. Even though I knew weight gain could only make matters worse, I kept eating and drinking because, at the moment, it was the only reliably enjoyable thing in my life. And even though I knew that exercise would make me feel better, and it would reverse my weight gain, I simply didn't feel like putting in the effort. *"I'm already unhappy,"* I said to myself, *"Why make myself even more unhappy by going out into the cold and being uncomfortable?"*

I knew the right answer to my rhetorical question. But I rarely offered it. Within six months, I'd gained twelve pounds. This isn't all that much, but when my tummy was formerly flat and my jeans used to barely cling to my hipbones, it was a nightmare.

It was time to return to that place where I got my satisfaction from self-control, not from self-indulgence. The question was: how?

LOSING IT AFTER YOU'VE LOST IT

Do you know the phrase, "You can never go home again"? It refers to when you've left your hometown and gone out on your own for some length of time. Upon returning, you find that the town no longer feels like home. Except it's not the town that has changed, it's you.

I think it's the same in weight loss. When seeking motivation, it can be fruitless to try to "go home," to return to what worked long ago. You've changed inside, and you must find your motivation afresh. With me, for example, losing weight is no longer like it formerly was. It's no longer an instant change fueled by the adrenaline hit of discovering thinspo and by the euphoria of realizing that I actually can have self-control. In the beginning, I was just so curious to see what I could accomplish! Now, however, I no longer have all that excitement keeping me going. Instead, I have to look deep inside to find my motivation. I have to carefully and painstakingly peel away each bad habit, one by one, replacing it with a good habit. It requires a seriously focused effort.

I've also recognized that *attitude* is THE most important thing. What was it that spurred me on in the beginning? What provoked me to embrace something which I knew would be incredibly hard, something at which I had always before failed? It was a positive attitude of hope. Hope that maybe, *just maybe*, I could actually do it this time. I was in love with the idea of discovering the awesomeness of getting skinny, rather than merely hating my fat.

And therein lies the answer. We must stay POSITIVE about weight loss.

Think about it: if you're being negative about anything, it doesn't lift you up, it drags you down. Being negative about fat puts you in a place where your strongest temptations are harmful ones. In such moments, we're tempted to binge, to starve, to purge, to cut, or what have you. Yet none of us is tempted to do any of these when our minds are in sunny and cheerful places.

Such was my problem. I'd fallen into negative thinking about fat gain, instead of positive thinking about weight loss. When I got heavier, instead of thinking, *"Keep working hard, you're going to look and feel awesome once you're at your goal,"* I was thinking,

"CRAP, I'm fat! This sucks! I looked so much better when I was skinny." Instead of *"Keep on running this race!"* I was like, *"You mean I have to enter that damned race again?"*

Yes, my dear, you do. And you need to stay positive about it, or you won't have the courage to pick yourself up after you stumble and fall.

Thankfully, on days when I maintain a goal-oriented, positive manner of thinking, making the painful decisions actually feels *good.* I enjoy satisfaction from staying hungry just a little bit longer, from denying self, from that wonderful sense of being on top of the world that follows each moment of hard-won self control. However, on days when I'm negative, when I complain about my flab and the effort required to lose it, even such things as lacing up my running shoes and going to bed slightly hungry are simply too great a burden.

In the end, although I'm now fighting a different battle than I was when I first began, it's still the same war. The difference is only that I've become a more seasoned veteran. Instead of my challenge being to keep up with the brutal pace of Boot Camp, it is now to keep up my morale under the relentless weeks and months of combat.

So many times I've said "this is hard, but it's worth it." And yet I somehow still imagined it would eventually become completely natural for me, and not require any real effort. Long after ceasing to be fat, however, I can say with some authority: *it never gets truly easy.* It gets *easier,* of course, but never actually, in the long run, easy.

For those of us to whom skinny does not naturally come, staying skinny will never require anything less than a constant state of vigilance. For us, we must maintain a perpetual watch. Is this fair? It doesn't matter. What matters is that, for us, this is the only way.

And it is STILL Worth It.

You can do this

A | Nothing Fits!
(Questions, that is)

Project:
Write yourself a letter from the future skinny you.
Write another from the future fat you.
Choose which one you're going to meet.

It's time to address all the random questions that don't really belong anywhere else. Although they're random, they probably still apply to things you were wondering about. Here, we talk about targeting fat loss, diet pills, how frequently you should weigh yourself, which weight loss studies you should consider, the effects of smoking, how to get thigh gap, what to do about saggy skin and thinning hair, and more. Do stick around.

Most of my body looks fine, except for [that one irritating part]. How do I target fat loss?

One universal rule I've seen many times over the years is that you cannot make fat disappear from only a certain area. Your body decides where to store fat. You cannot lose stomach fat by doing sit-ups, arm flab by working out your arms, thigh fat by doing leg exercises, or drinking any kind of tea to remove fat from X body part.

The only way to get rid of fat from one area is simply by losing fat in general. While you may like your body in every area except one, you have to lose weight all over for that one spot to subside. This is good and bad: if you really, truly do have excess fat *only* in that one area, it should rapidly begin to disappear. However, if you, like almost everybody, have a little excess elsewhere, you are going to lose some of the other fat, too, making it seem like it is taking *forever* to lose the fat from the one place you are targeting. Don't fight it, but just realize that you are going to look better everywhere, not just that one place.

In my experience, as I dropped the pounds, I noticed the fat did not come off uniformly. I first noticed it leaving my face and thighs. Next, my pants fit a little looser. Then my shirts fit looser in the chest. At one time, I saw the number going down on the scale for several days, but the pair of jeans I was trying to fit into simply wouldn't fit any looser. It turns out my stomach fat was standing fast, but I was losing fat from my arms and butt. Even my wrists and fingers have gotten much slimmer. Although I'd rather all the fat come off my stomach, thighs, and face before coming off anywhere else, it just doesn't happen that way. I'm just glad it came off at all. I still feel like a success. I had to be more patient than I would have liked, but it's been a small price to pay.

Diet pills. Yea or nay?

Pills are temporary. Attitude is forever.

Several times in my past, I took various diet pills, including some pretty hardcore stuff that you can't buy in America (hey, I heard it increased your metabolism and decreased your appetite—and I was desperate). Each time, they did nothing for my weight loss, because what I really needed was to stop eating so much. All they did was to make me slightly more broke and, in one case, make me feel like a thousand butterflies were seeking to burst forth from my chest. Looks romantic in print, feels like crap in real life.

Diet pills are a bad way to go. They're just an example of hoping someone else will solve your problems, an ineffective mentality for permanent weight loss. The pills merely distract you from the fact that the food you choose to put in your own mouth is what makes you the size you are.

Long-term weight loss requires a healthy-eating mindset, not a pill-taking mindset. It's important to learn how to eat properly, rather than focusing just on the immediate weight loss itself. To buy pills is to spend a bunch of money on something that 'doesn't actually take care of any nutritional needs. Wouldn't it be so much better to spend that same money on natural and nutritious foods?

I heard it's best to avoid weighing yourself daily, because the fluctuations will just discourage and frustrate you.

I weigh myself every day, always first thing in the morning after using the bathroom but before eating or drinking. That is the best way to avoid fluctuations. Weighing yourself at other times means you have undigested food and unprocessed water making your number higher. And you know higher numbers are *always* discouraging.

I'm not the only one who thinks this is a good idea. In a famous massive study of people who lost at least 30 pounds and kept it off for a year or longer, daily weighing was the *single most common factor*. Daily weighing alerts you to how your body is responding to your behavior. It actually rocks.

Let me give you an example. Let's say you weigh yourself every Sunday, but not at any other time during the week. You choose this because you heard it's bad to weigh yourself daily. The idea is, after a whole week of good self-control, you will have lost weight, right?

But what if on Saturday, you ate some particularly salty food? *Bam!* Your weight will be higher Sunday, because you're retaining water. You're not actually fatter; in fact, you may have lost fat! But you are heavier and puffier and therefore feel like a failure, and are tempted to give up altogether.

It gets worse. What if, one week ago, you happened to get in a ton of exercise the day before you weighed yourself, but this week, you had a couple of exercise-free days before you weighed in? Your weight from last time will be your *dehydrated* weight, and therefore unnaturally low, but your weight this week will be what you weigh after you have replenished your body's fluids. You might think you gained weight when you actually did not.

The point is, weighing yourself after long durations makes you more likely to think things are not working *at all* if you don't see the number you were hoping for. Daily weighing, however, allows you to ignore the little fluctuations. It teaches you that other factors than fat can account for such fluctuations. Seriously, I've had days where I've eaten fewer than 800 calories, *and* exercised, but my weight still went up the next day. That's not real! Daily weighing lets you follow the general *trend* of your weight, and it teaches you how your body responds to differing amounts of food and exercise.

All that said, if you are the kind of person who *really* gets down on yourself any time you see a higher number on the scale, you may want to throw out your scale entirely and start using another form of measurement instead. Taking body measurements with a tape measure, or even seeing how close you are to fitting into your pair of "goal jeans," is also perfectly valid.

I want a thigh gap! I've been working out and getting skinny, but still no gap. How do I get it?

Thigh gap is *not* just a factor of skinny. It involves a whole mixture of skinniness, age, and genetics. Some stockier girls have it, some really skinny girls don't. Young girls are less likely to have it than are their fully developed future selves. It also involves your skeletal build and your body's preference to store fat in your thighs or in other places. Really, this question is almost like asking, "How do I get born with blue eyes?"

So, how *do* you work on getting a thigh gap?
1. Be completely developed, puberty-wise.
2. Have an certain genetic makeup.
3. Lose weight.
4. Combine all of the above.

If you're young, wait for #1. If you're overweight, work on #3 (but please don't become unhealthy for such an unimportant goal!). And #2 is impossible to change, so please don't try to be somebody you're not.

I'm shedding tons of weight, and I fear my skin will become saggy and gross. How do I prevent this?

I highly doubt that will happen. It often takes a weight loss of over a hundred pounds before that becomes an issue. Even if your skin does become a little loose, it should return to a nice, taut, firm condition after a few months at your new weight.

If all else fails, just try to accept that this is what they call "a nice problem to have." It's still better (and better for you) than being fat is.

What about my shrinking boobs?

They may become smaller, but fear not: when you lose weight, you lose only fat from your chest, not breast tissue. They won't completely disappear no matter how skinny you get. Give them time, and they will perk back up as the skin around them grows firmer. Actually, after that happens, they should also sag less than they previously did, which you must admit is a bonus.

Consider also—and I'm being serious here—they're just boobs. Would you *really* rather be bigger just so they are?

I hear smoking reduces your appetite. I could really use that.

You've already heard all the preaching on why you shouldn't smoke. Let's bypass all that and focus only on weight loss.

Whether or not smoking helps in the short term, remember that eating less and exercising at least a little bit is the *only viable way* to lose weight and keep it off. Everything else, including smoking, is either temporary, or potentially deadly, or both.

My hair is thinning out as I'm eating less. Is this normal?

Whoa, hold on! This is a problem! Hair loss is common amongst people who are *malnourished!* It could be a sign that your body is not getting the nutrients you need. I recommend you immediately increase your intake of *healthful*, nutrient-dense foods. If that doesn't have an immediate effect, it's time to see your doctor, as you may have a serious condition requiring medical treatment.

A scientific study shows that eating less [meat / fat / carbs / whatever] is linked to weight loss. Thoughts?

Ah, the ever-present "scientific study". Almost everything has been recommended at one time or another, including the opposite of everything that was formerly recommended. The one thing I do know is that *eating less of everything* is a proven method. It's the only one I use.

Occasionally, I skip a meal entirely. Is that wrong?

I once had a conversation with a 60-year-old man. He was in good shape but did no exercise other than regular golfing. He mentioned that the way he stayed in shape was by skipping dinner every night. He had done this for years. If he didn't go to bed hungry, he said, he would gain weight.

At the time, I thought he was nuts. But he did what worked for him. He ate big American breakfasts with eggs, bacon, and toast, plus full-sized lunches of whatever he wanted to eat, but he simply made the choice to stop there. And it worked for him for decades.

It's weird how, if a young woman did the same thing, she would be accused of having an ED, yet this man would probably be praised for his "old fashioned wisdom." Funny world we live in.

The point is: do what works for you. Eating disorders are rooted in your opinion of your body, not in what others say about your diet.

B | How to Run

It's easier to run when you're skinny. It's easier to be skinny when you run.

"How to Run" is definitely an ambitious title for such a tiny chapter. I could have called it "How I Became a Runner," but the funny thing is, about a year and a half after I wrote the following advice and published it online, the Associated Press put out a major news article containing advice from an expert saying almost exactly the same thing! Seriously, it was like he was summarizing my old article. This being the case, I feel pretty good about presenting you with what is now apparently "expert" advice.

This chapter's format is a little different. Rather than giving you a polished, "final" version, I'm including my article as it originally appeared online (starting when I was about ten weeks into my journey), followed by the individual updates I made to it as I learned new things about running over the months.

MONTH ONE: GETTING STARTED

Running, seemingly more than any other exercise, burns serious calories and is one of the few things that genuinely does "rev up" your metabolism. There is probably no better exercise if you need the pounds to come off, *pronto*. As an added bonus, it's cheap to do, it's among the safer sports, it allows you to catch some scenery, and you can do it anywhere.

I've pretty much hated running, and been quite bad at it, forever. Nevertheless, I chose to start running because I know it really works at getting a person in shape. Good news: as I have gotten more in shape, running has gotten *much* easier, and now some days I actually enjoy it! Really, often I just set out running, and for the first little while I get this feeling of "*Wow, I'm really flying effortlessly along!*" That feeling is amazing.

Want to similarly feel amazing? Here's how:

Start with what you can do—and just do it.

If you need to run one minute and then walk two minutes to catch your breath, then run another minute and walk two more ... do it! That's how I started. Soon you're able to run two and walk one. Then you can run five and walk one. And so on. Right now—and I still need to lose quite a bit of weight—I can run more than twenty minutes before needing to walk.

Try to run just a little farther each time.

This is an awesome and interesting way to increase your ability. If you regularly run a certain road or path, try to run a little farther than you ran last time before you turn around. If you do a loop in the city or suburbs, try to run one more block than you did the previous time before making your turn. If you time yourself, try to last one minute longer than last time before stopping. If you run a track, aim to complete one extra lap each time you head out. It's fun to see yourself improving, and it helps make you better.

Alternately, try to run a little faster.

I often run a local scenic loop of 1.75 miles. I time myself and try to make sure that each time is just a little bit faster than the last, even if by only a few seconds. Seeing the improvement in time makes it much more rewarding and motivating than just saying, "Yeah, so I ran it again ... yawn."

If at all possible, find a running partner.

You will run virtually twice as far with a partner, because you won't want to be the first one to stop. It is actually *easier* to keep running this way. Plus, you can talk a little in between huffs and puffs, which distracts you from what might otherwise be tedium. Talking while running also increases the aerobic workout you get from the run, and it makes the time go by faster.

Get the right shoes.

Are you an over-pronator, under-pronator, or neutral? If you don't know the answer to this question, you might be wearing the wrong shoes and therefore hurting yourself. You would also be making your running harder than it needs to be. Go to an actual running store (NOT just a general sporting goods store or shoe store) and have them examine your stride and the shape of your arch. They will recommend the best kind of shoe for your body. Any of the big name running shoes is fine as long as you get the shoe that has the right features for your feet. Each brand fits differently, too, so don't forget to try different models. Finally, spend some money. A few extra dollars for high quality shoes is a tiny price to pay to avoid injury! I speak from experience.

Give yourself rest, especially in the beginning when you are just getting into running.

You can't run several days in a row without your body complaining. Especially when you are just starting out, your muscles will be sore in places you didn't know you had muscles, including tiny little support muscles around your ankles and feet, or in your neck, shoulders, and, of course, the big muscles in your legs. Let your body heal and strengthen by giving it a day or two of rest before you work out again. When you stop feeling sore the following day is when you no longer need to rest in between runs. Even then, don't exercise more than five or six days a week without giving your body rest, or you may be flirting with injury.

Happy trails!

MONTH TWO: HOW COOL IT CAN GET

Although I previously mentioned being able to run for up to twenty minutes without walking, which I thought was pretty amazing, I recently discovered something even *more* amazing! I accidentally found myself at the point where I realized I didn't have to stop at *all*.

Runs used to always get noticeably harder the longer into

them I was, and often, I would say to myself, *"I'm getting tired. I'm going to walk."* Late into a run, I would have to stop to walk every five minutes.

The other day, however, I set out for an extra long run, planning to run about four miles. Around forty minutes into my run, I had already stopped to walk a couple of times, and I was about to walk again out of habit. But for some reason, the idea popped up, *"I guess this isn't actually killing me. Maybe I can keep running."* I *did* keep running—for an additional 22 minutes—and set a new personal record: 5.1 miles, my longest run ever! Even then, I didn't actually need to stop; it was merely time to go home.

The point here is: keep on running, and you will get to the place where your heart and lungs are strong enough that they can more than keep up. Since realizing this, I have purposefully set longer and longer goals for myself each time I've run. The strangest thing is: the longer of a goal I set, the easier of a time I have running! This reveals that, often, *"tired" is all in your head.*

Here's what I mean: A few weeks after the above-mentioned 5.1-mile run, I set another new record, running 6.6 miles and only stopping to walk *twice.* Later, I shattered that record, running 8.5 miles. That's a third of a marathon! The best part was, the first *seven* miles of the 8.5-mile run were easier than was the *entire* 6.6-mile run! It's not that I was in better shape, it's that, in my mind, when miles five and six rolled around, instead of thinking, *"OMG this is a long run, but it's almost over,"* I was thinking, *"Six miles down? Okay then, two and a half more to go."* For some reason, since I knew I had to keep it up for a while longer, it's like my brain didn't allow me to start thinking, *"Quit soon,"* and that provided me with actual physical energy.

Note on increasing speed

Now that I've become able to run longer without stopping, I wondered how to improve my speed (if I'm going to enter a half marathon—yes, that is my goal—I want to cross the finish line before they pack up and go home). I actually picked up a running magazine at the bookstore (those magazines always used to seem like they were in a foreign language) and I read about how to get better at long runs. The article said to try interval training: go hard for two minutes, then jog for two minutes, go hard for two, jog two, etc. Apparently, this is supposed to train your body to realize that it has more to give, even when it's tired.

I tried it recently. It was actually really cool! Although the fast running moments were hard, I didn't feel like I was going to die, and I felt quite speedy! My head actually swelled a little when I blasted past walkers while I was charging full speed ahead. The slower moments were really great, allowing me to catch my breath. Added bonus: my usual loop, which I'd never run faster than 17:30 before, I finished in an even 16:30! Not only is the interval training supposed to make me faster generally, It's already making me faster right now! Highly recommended.

MONTH THREE: WHAT IS HAPPENING?

Okay, I keep learning about running as I do it more! These days, I'm actually starting to LIKE running! I can't believe it! I mean, I still don't "like" running the way you like a hobby or pastime, but I do find myself getting excited about running. This is not so much because the running is *fun* (let's face it: it's still no picnic) but because getting *good* at running *is* fun! Better than fun, getting good at running is *elating*.

Growing up, I was usually the worst runner in my class. But today, I actually went to a local running store and inquired about how to sign up for a half marathon. This weekend, weather permitting, I plan to see if I can make it around a scenic trail over ten miles long. I have butterflies in my stomach thinking about it. Not because I'm scared to try but because *I think I might actually be able to do it!* Me, the fatso!

I just want to cry, this is so wonderful and marvelous to contemplate. It's like I'm the character in a rags-to-riches fairy tale, only it's better than that because *riches couldn't make me as happy as becoming skinny is making me.*

MONTH FOUR: DAY OF RECKONING

[I ran the half marathon! But you already know that story, so I won't repeat it here.]

MONTH FIVE: OOPS!

I just ran 35 minutes and actually *forgot* to walk! This makes me laugh happy laughter.

MONTH SIX: I SURRENDER!

Okay, I give in! I actually *like* running now. As in, I find myself in the mood to do it. It makes me happy. I enjoy watching the scenery go by. I enjoy feeling like I can do it and not die. I enjoy knowing that I'm burning hundreds of calories each time I head out. I enjoy getting all that air and sun (and even rain). I enjoy when strangers see me out running and have no idea that I haven't always done this. I enjoy telling people that I went for a "short" run of "only" four miles. I enjoy that I have been given new life. I am amazed. This is SO cool.

C | Food and Drink (I Get It: Eat Small— but What Foods, and How?)

Light eating cookbooks are no solution to heavy eating habits.

Following recipes isn't how I lost weight. Still, I do have a few ideas which should help. Just be sure to do your homework to find out what foods are both enjoyable to you and nutrient-dense. Each of us has our own best way of eating. I recommend you experiment to find what works for you and what you can make into a long-term habit.

How do you find the time to make healthful meals?

There's no need to spend time in the kitchen making fancy "low calorie" meals. You can totally do this on the fly if you want to. But it's *much* better if you at least *plan* your intake somewhat in advance, else you will sometimes find yourself hungry and food-less, approaching the only food source around, stuck between ordering garbage or crap. Not a good place.

As for me, I haven't spent any *more* time making meals than I used to. I just substitute good food for bad. In the past, I bought low-calorie cookbooks and tried to make meals from them, but it was just too much hassle. Today, I simply eat *less*. It seems unnatural at first—but then you realize it was actually the large portions you were previously eating that were "unnatural". A simple modification to the hedonistic portions we tend to eat is all it takes.

I find it hard to get in my eight glasses of water every day.

You poor thing! There's no need! The "eight glasses of water a day" mantra is nonsense. I know, I know, you've heard it thousands of times. But that doesn't make it true. The reason we keep hearing it is because people have twisted the findings of an ancient study which got repeated so much that it has snowballed into this huge thing that "everybody knows" but which is false.

The actual study in question found that our bodies need 1 milliliter of water for every calorie consumed. If you use the 2000-calories-per-day-diet (eek!) as your guide, that corresponds to 2000 milliliters of water, or eight 8-oz glasses. But the same study ALSO said (and almost everyone leaves this part out!!) that *you get most of the water you need from the foods you consume*—which consist mostly of, believe it or not, WATER.[18]

I feel so sorry for these people trying to drink a gallon of water a day, running to the bathroom every 30 minutes. It's tragically superfluous. Go ahead and drink plenty of water if you want to, just don't beat yourself up for not cramming it into yourself simply because someone distorted a study's findings. Stay hydrated, but stay sane.

Should I cut out meat?

I don't want to get into the arguments behind the subject of meat eating (you do know that humans cannot live without certain vitamins that are naturally found *only in meat*, right?), but I wanted to bring up the weight-loss implications of it. I find that there tend to be two kinds of people who go meat-free:

1. Those who *lose* weight when they stop eating meat.
2. Those who *gain* weight when they stop eating meat.

I am wholly convinced that the people who lose weight when they stop eating meat do so simply because they are finally *watching what they put in their mouths*, not because meat was making them fat. *Just being aware of what you eat* (as a new vegetarian always is) can be enough for you to abandon the mindless bad habits you had before, thus resulting in weight loss.[19]

The people who *gain* weight—and this happens a lot—gain weight, it seems, because they make up for the absence of meat in their diets with too many carbs (which screws with your insulin production and fat absorption, causing you to pack on the pounds) or with too much splurging on other foods, seeking to satisfy the unfulfilled meat cravings.

My proposal: why not just imitate the first group, and *pay at-*

---

[18] Even a potato, for example, consists of 80% water. Look it up yourself if you like.
[19] I'm convinced that this is why every diet out there "works" for the first little while.

tention to what you eat, without resorting to a diet which leaves you constantly craving? Get the nutrients you need, reap the benefits, shed the pounds.

You're at a restaurant with friends or family. What do you do?

I eat what I want, but in small amounts. I try not to order a whole meal, but only a side dish, or a salad, or I share an entrée with someone. Modern restaurant portions are outrageous, and a single dish often has more calories than your entire daily need. You can eat far less than that and still enjoy being out. Think of the menu as a minefield and tread carefully.

As for ordering something to drink: when dining out, I still want to enjoy myself. It's one thing to watch calories, but I don't want to hate my life. I order something I'll enjoy, but I'm *very* mindful that many drinks contain empty calories, and usually little to no nutritional value. Unsweetened iced tea is awesome, as is coffee (watch out for sugar and cream calories). I also love sparkling water with a wedge of lime. Zero calories, but it tastes like a soda. Actual sodas, however: never. They're simply not worth the damage they do.

If we're drinking alcohol, I'll have wine or beer if I can afford the calories that day, because sometimes they just go SO perfectly with the meal. I try to avoid cocktails, however, because the stuff they mix the drinks with is almost always *heavily* sugared.

A couple more tips:

- Would you pay money to lose weight? Sure you would. So don't worry if you pay for food that you don't finish. Just because something shows up on your plate doesn't mean you have to eat it. When you jump on the scale next morning, it will have been worth the price.

- If you can't make do with just a small dish, ask for a takeaway box *before* you tear into your meal. Put in half, then just eat what remains. If that is too weird for the people you're with, try as hard as you can to leave enough on your plate that you can ask for a box after. Yes, it's very hard to stop. Those delicious bites are very attractive. But skinny is more attractive.

How do you survive an all-you-can-eat buffet?

It amazes me that the phrase "All You Can Eat" used to be attractive to me, not abhorrent! Nonetheless, I have attended several all-you-can-eat events and been okay, so long as certain precautions are taken. You don't want to simply skip eating, but you don't want to undo your hard work, either. Here is how I recommend approaching the situation:

- Use the smallest plate you can find.
- Decide up front that you are NOT going back for seconds.
- DON'T try every item; choose only the foods you would cry about later if you missed them.
- Take only one or two forkfuls of each of those foods.
- Load up on vegetables as much as possible, even though you really crave the other stuff. Your conscience will thank you later.
- If at a social event, try to spend as much time as possible standing around talking, not sitting down to tear into your meal. Simply hold your plate and talk. Or set it down next to you and talk. Just talk.
- Hold a drink while you're chatting. People won't notice you're not eating because it always looks like you're about to take a sip from your glass.
- Take extra small bites so it takes longer to eat.
- Once you've finished your plate and you are on the verge of going psycho because you so badly want to go back for seconds, you can ignore your "no seconds" rule and treat yourself to ONE bite each of TWO yummy things.
- *Dessert*: since you've controlled yourself, you can reward yourself. Cut yourself a tiny slice, or take only half of a cookie, or otherwise give yourself a portion that is a quarter the size of what everyone else is eating. You will still enjoy it as much as you would have enjoyed a huge serving. Plus, dessert is the one thing you can publicly skimp on without others objecting.
- *Drinks*: watch those empty calories. You want coffee, unsweetened iced tea, water. If you're drinking alcohol, realize that it has a lot of calories, and you should con-

sider it a replacement for some of the extra food that you are now NOT going to eat because of those calories.

Finally, if you blow it and wind up overeating: RELAX. The only way to lose weight and keep it off is to have a long term goal. Don't let this single setback cause you to lose sight of that. At least you tried—how many others weren't even trying to go easy on the food? You are still on the right path. You are still learning how to succeed. You are not a failure, you are a work in progress. You blew it for ONE DAY. Now it will take you ONE DAY LONGER to reach your goal. That's not so bad.

An article in a health magazine told me to eat / not eat X.

I've read a hundred health magazines over the years. One thing I notice is that they're ALWAYS changing their minds about what foods to eat or avoid. It makes sense: the magazines wouldn't exactly fly off the shelves if their covers blazed, *"Lose Weight by Eating the Same Foods We Told You About Six Months Ago!"*

Read health magazines for inspiration and for general information, but don't hang off of every last word they print.

Help! I have no idea what to eat. How do I know what's nutritious?

Learning this does require a little research on your part. Thankfully, that information is everywhere, and it's free (so enjoy doing your homework).

Perhaps the best advice I've received is to try to eat foods as closely as possible to their natural state. The less processed, the better. I think we should be *really* wary of ingesting any "food" that can sit for months on a shelf without spoiling.

Also, I don't eat fast food. Like, ever.

What?!? Don't you miss eating fast food?

Of course I do. I miss it about as much as I miss being fat.

Would it still be okay if I had fast food in small portions?

It shouldn't be a problem. I don't think there is any food that is particularly "evil". Keep the amounts small and the rest should take care of itself. I think that ice cream, chips—heck, even deep-fried butter—are all okay, as long as they're eaten in small amounts. I don't believe in "diets" where you're supposed to succeed by completely cutting out such-and-such a thing.

That said, if you can eat a salad instead of a burger, yeah, that will help.[20]

My cafeteria offers vegetarian dishes, but I wonder if they're any better for me.

Vegetarians often get stuck with pasta choices, or something similarly filling but starchy. If that's the case, be careful, because that's a lot of high-carb intake. Make sure your "vegetarian" meal includes a lot of actual *vegetables*, else it may actually be worse for you than the other options are.

Do you ever get cravings for fatty foods, and do you give into them?

Rich foods, sure, like cheese, *pâté*, and other fine foods, just not fried chicken, pizza, burgers, and so on. If I'm going to eat something high in calories, it has to be worth it. And I eat small portions only.

However, if you are experiencing withdrawal symptoms and fear that you will go crazy if you don't get some of that deep-fried deliciousness, make sure that you eat only the smallest amount you can. A few bites should be enough to scratch that itch. Allow yourself to experience happiness that you stopped, not regret that you started.

I don't want to completely give up alcohol. How can I lose weight while still going to parties?

Alcohol slows the weight loss, but certainly doesn't stop it. However, it's empty calories, and it slows your metabolism until after your body has burned off the alcohol, so you must be

---

[20] So long as it's a good salad, not one of those 1500-calorie monstrosities that many restaurants serve.

careful.

If I know I'm going to drink on a certain night, I try to "earn" my alcohol by exercising that afternoon. And because I know alcohol really messes with my self control, and I sometimes wind up eating too much as a result, I am VERY careful to make up my mind beforehand that I will NOT indulge at the party in any more food than usual. It requires real vigilance.

As long as you go to the party with the mindset, "I will not eat crap food," you should be able to *avoid* gaining weight. Just bear in mind you're not exactly going to *lose* much weight, either.

Pretty much all that my friends want to do is go out every night and drink / eat. How can I lose the weight and not the friends?

If I were to try to distill it all into a single "formula," I'd offer: More drinks = harder to say no to food = easier to hate yourself later, whereas more self-control = guaranteed pleasure with how you behaved.

Isn't pleasure the reason you go out in the first place? Food and drink give only shallow pleasure. Knowing you're healthy and liking how you look gives profound joy.

Unfortunately, you can achieve such joy only by denying short-term indulgences in favor of long-term satisfaction. Promise yourself you will eat only the tiniest of portions, no matter what your friends are eating. If they bug you about it, tell them you're teaching yourself how to eat more healthily. If they persist in pestering you, tell them *"This is something I need to do for ME."* If they're true friends, they'll back off.

What do you think of 100-calorie snack packs?

I'm torn between two opinions:

1. They are awesome because they have enough food in them to take away your hunger without scuttling your intake plans.
2. They are crap because they are usually highly processed food loaded with carbs and/or salt.

Is milk a good drink?

You asked the right person! Seriously, I'm a recovering milkaholic.

Milk does have protein and calcium, among other good nutrients, and sometimes it's exactly what you crave. In those moments, go for it, but you do have to count it as intake (water, on the other hand, is always a freebie). A single small glass of milk contains over 100 calories, and it probably won't leave you feeling as satisfied as if you'd had the same number of calories' worth of nutritious food. But it's your call.

Water is so boring!

I found a way to make water *delicious*, and I mean so delicious you crave it.

I once spent a day at a really posh spa, and their icy jugs of water contained slices of lemons and, oddly, cucumber. Oh my gosh, I swear I *binged on water* that day! If you've never tried the combination, you *must!* I can't even describe how much better it tastes than it sounds (and I don't think it sounds bad). I make it at home by combining a large bottle of spring water with two thin slices of lemon and five slices of cucumber (you can play with the ratio to get the flavor you prefer). It's Heaven in a glass.

Other fruit and herb combinations (hello, mint leaves!) can be just as heavenly. Try some out!

Can I drink diet sodas? They contain no calories.

I would be cautious with diet sodas. Some people say they're worse for you than sugary sodas are, and that they actually cause your body to store fat. I don't know how true that is, but I do have an interesting personal experience I'd like to share.

Months after cutting out diet sodas and allowing my body to purge itself of all the chemicals from them, I found myself from time to time wanting a cold drink, and I would have access only to water or soft drinks. Bored with water and unwilling to drink sugar, I would grab a diet soda. But half an hour later, I would find myself just feeling so … *bad*. Every time, I'd feel weary, my head would be fuzzy, and I'd want little else but to take a nap. I'm convinced that it was the artificial sweetener chemicals that did it. Moreover, my weight loss seemed to slow on the days I drank that stuff.

Point is, if you can avoid diet sodas, I'm sure you'll be better off. If you still crave tiny bubbles in your drinks, I recommend the naturally fruit-flavored sparkling waters that are out there. They're not sweetened, but the fruit flavor tricks you into thinking they are. Super refreshing and guilt-free.

Do you completely abstain from any particular foods?

I definitely stay away from the usual suspects (burgers, pizza, anything deep-fried, frozen blended coffee drinks, chips, sodas, etc). But if I'm in a situation where those are the only choices I have, I just make sure to eat a VERY small portion, perhaps just one slice of pizza, and the smallest one I can find.

What foods meet your nutritional needs, and fill you up, and are also low in calories?

Typically, things with lots of fiber (awesome lists of high-fiber foods are easily found online), and lots of salads with not too much cheese or dressing. For protein, I like low-fat string cheese, as well as eggs, turkey, and so on. I also take a multi-vitamin (*really* important when you're reducing calories, because you're also reducing nutrients).

I don't really eat any "magic" things. I eat "normal" food, just less of it. I also find that the more healthful the food, the more of it I can eat for the same number of calories. The other night, for example, I ate a homemade vegetable stew. I filled up for next to no calories, and I got tons of lovely nutrients.

I love big, greasy breakfasts, but I know I need to make a change. Any ideas for low-calorie but filling breakfasts?

They say breakfast is the most important meal of the day. I agree, but in what is probably the opposite way from what you've heard. Instead of eating a big breakfast to help make it through the day, I eat a tiny breakfast to set the stage for a day of good eating.

I find in general that I will be hungry a few hours after breakfast no matter how much I eat, *unless* I have shrunk my stomach by making *every* meal small, *every* day. Nowadays I can eat a single soft-boiled egg, wash it down with tea or coffee, and be good until lunchtime. Seriously. But that's because I've shrunk my stomach by avoiding bingeing.

Here are a few other good breakkie ideas that work for me:

- The best low-calorie, filling breakfast ever: liquid eggs scrambled together with onions and tomatoes (or spinach). It's much like eating a traditional omelet, yet it's super low in calories and super high in protein. Plus, you get vegetables! This can be very filling and nutritious and, if you keep the portion reasonable (and use a cooking spray, not butter or oil), it's barely over 100 calories. Also, if it's what you really crave, you could add a slice of bacon for only about 60 calories more.

- Oatmeal (small portion, perhaps half a cup before cooking—don't worry, it expands a lot when cooking) with a dash of salt (which will make it taste almost as if you'd added butter). I add no sugar, only a small teaspoon of natural nut butter (I like roasted almond butter, but you can use natural peanut butter or, for a more exotic taste, tahini). Pour a little milk over the top and enjoy! 125–200 calories depending on how easy you go on the nut butter.

- A piece of fruit and a portion of string cheese. It's filling, and the cheese makes the fruit go down better. About 100+ calories.

- A vegetarian breakfast sausage (or two). Not super filling, but satisfying and it's indulgent-feeling in those moments when you crave that greasy traditional breakfast. 80-160 calories.

What about the rest of the day?

I don't like to plan everything in advance, so I try simply to keep good food around, and I refuse to buy bad stuff that I'll be tempted to snack on.

Lunch: I sometimes make a small sandwich with meat and sliced cucumbers. As a spread I use hummus instead of mayo (if you really want to go low-cal—and can handle the taste—use only mustard).

I also really love making my own lettuce wraps (I call them "lettuce canoes" because I use long romaine lettuce spears and that's what the shape reminds me of): just take a big piece of lettuce and put some lean protein on it. Roll and munch! For convenience's sake, I use pre-cooked seasoned chicken already sliced into small pieces.

Dinner. I love eating giant homemade salads for dinner. I can eat almost as much as I want, and it provides a zillion nutrients I would otherwise miss out on. I make my salads purposefully to get *tons* of vegetables, not merely lettuce and dressing. If not in the mood for salad, I'll have a portion of meat with some kind of vegetable. I avoid rice, bread, noodles, and so on, because they're super calorie-dense and not at all nutrient-dense.

Describe a typical day from when you were still losing weight?

Just for you, I recorded my intake one day when I was working on losing weight:

- Breakfast: oatmeal with 1 tbsp fresh cranberry sauce and milk, unsweetened tea with milk. 150 cal (plus a multivitamin washed down with a swig of milk, 20 cal).
- Morning snack: miniature high-fiber bran muffin. 80 cal.
- Late lunch: turkey sandwich made with one slice of 45-calorie bread, lots of turkey, a little avocado. 150 cal.
- Dinner: chicken breast (I removed most but not all of the skin), a tiny bit of cranberry sauce (weird to have it twice in one day, but it's what I had available), and a tomato-eggplant dish I got at the store. 400 cal.
- TOTAL: 800 calories.

This was a good day. As you can see, I got to eat often. Now before anyone gets upset that this isn't enough nutrients, please remember that this was just one day, and other days I consumed more vegetables (and, often, more calories). Also, eating like this was temporary: once I hit my goal, I added to my everyday intake.

SUMMARY

This is not a ton of ideas, but I never intended for this to become a cookbook. I obviously eat far more things than I describe here, but really, none of that matters, because you need to find what works for you. You get the idea: eat natural foods, eat small amounts, and try to keep it to foods you'd be proud to be seen eating. What will follow is a body that you are proud to be seen in.

D | The 1200-Calorie Myth

It's going to be hard either way, so take your pick:
the hard-to-implement path or the hard-to-live-with-yourself-afterwards
path.

I've often faced ridicule from people who have heard that 1200 calories is the minimum amount of food that a woman can eat without malnourishing herself. In my mind and my heart, and based on my own experiences, I've known that this is untrue. I consistently ate less than 1200 calories a day, month after month, while keeping in perfect health. So who is right? Bothered by this question, I set out to put this argument to rest and determine the answer.

As you already read on page 45, the 1200-calorie recommendation is a *general* recommendation, which takes into account the foods that *average* people *often* eat. This is what the public health officials have to deal with when they issue their guidelines. As you can imagine, it's far easier for the policymakers to enshrine a "golden number" of calories to eat than it is for them to actually educate people on *which* kinds of calories to eat. Hence, the 1200-calorie compromise. 1200 calories is a doable amount for the "average" person, and it is a low enough target that most people serious about losing weight can achieve it without depriving themselves of essential nutrients.

But what if someone set out to choose *better* foods than the "average" person eats? What if she chose foods which provide the *same* amount of essential nutrients, yet are *lower* in calories? This is what I have done, and I think the results speak for themselves.

Regardless, let's fully illuminate this principle by considering a day in the life of two women who decided to make the changes required to lose the weight. One did it the "right" way, the other the "wrong" way. They both lost weight, but one went about things in a far healthier fashion.

AVERAGE WOMAN'S DAY OF WEIGHT LOSS

Average Woman needs to lose weight. She has heard from her doctor and the mainstream media that it's a good idea to "reduce" her intake. She has heard that she needs to go easy on high-fat and sugary foods, and that a 1200-calorie diet is recommended for people in her position. She dutifully sets out to change her lifestyle. Her goal is to obtain that healthy and svelte figure that has been eluding her for so long. Here's what she eats:

Breakfast

A "bowl" of cereal with milk. Average Woman keeps the amount of cereal down to the official "serving" size of 3/4 of a cup, or barely half a dozen spoonfuls.[21] Moments later, on her way to work, Average Woman stops at the coffee shop and picks up a 12-ounce latté (unsweetened—gotta watch those calories!).

Calories: 350. Protein: 12g. Fresh produce: none.

Lunch

Average Woman is ravenously hungry, as her tiny breakfast of simple carbs and milk digested hours ago. She didn't have time to pack a lunch today, so she heads for the most convenient option, the local fast food joint. She orders a small fried chicken sandwich (chicken is supposed to be better for you than beef) and a small order of fries (they're too hard to resist, but at least the small size appeases her cravings). To drink, Average Woman orders a diet soda.

Calories: 590. Protein: 15g. Fresh produce: a leaf of lettuce.

---

[21] Tell the truth: you *know* you can't eat such a small "serving" of breakfast cereal. But let's pretend Average Woman is stronger than you are.

Dinner

Tonight is Average Woman's night to meet with friends for dinner at their favorite restaurant. Feeling guilty about eating fries at lunch and for not eating enough vegetables, she orders a Caesar salad with grilled chicken. Conscious of her daily intake, she eats only half. She washes it down with water while everyone around her has sugary soft drinks and alcoholic beverages. She wishes she could join them, but she knows she needs to do this right if she's going to lose the weight.

Calories: 350. Protein: 28g. Fresh produce: a fair amount of lettuce.

At the end of the day:

Today, Average Woman exercised amazing restraint! She didn't eat perfectly, but she mostly stuck to her plan and ate a *very* sensible amount. Her doctor and the media have done their job, as has she.

Calories: 1240. Almost perfect! She flirted with the bottom range of the officially-sanctioned diet, but she didn't fall into the "unhealthy" range!

Protein: 53g. Awesome, considering the RDA (recommended daily amount) is 56g.

Fresh produce: lots of lettuce! Not a lot of nutrients, but at least it's green.

SKINNY WOMAN'S DAY OF WEIGHT LOSS

Next, let's picture someone who has read this book (let's call her "Skinny Woman"). She knows the usual recommendations are fine and all, but she feels like she can do better.

Breakfast

Two eggs scrambled with green onions, tomatoes, and cilantro; coffee with sugar (not *all* indulgences need be forsaken).

Calories: 200. Protein: 12g. Fresh produce: some.

Lunch

Skinny woman is hungry, but manageably so, because her breakfast of all natural foods took its time digesting and it provided her with energy all morning. She pulls out the lunch she made for herself this morning (in less time than it would now take her to get her lunch from the fast-food restaurant down the street): half of a ham and turkey sandwich with a little mustard, mayo, cucumber, and lettuce.

Calories: 200. Protein: 14g. Fresh produce: again, some

Afternoon Snack

Suffering from that age-old enemy of productivity, the Mid-Afternoon Slump, and also pretty hungry after eating only 400 calories so far, Skinny woman reaches into her bag and pulls out an orange that she brought with her in case of emergency. It's currently an emergency, so down the hatch it goes.

Calories: 60. Protein: 1g. Fresh produce: nothing but.

Dinner

Skinny Woman also eats out tonight, at a gathering at a friend's place. They are serving grilled marinated chicken breasts with Greek salad and rice. Skinny Woman enjoys some chicken and a generous portion of salad, but skips the rice.

Calories: 400. Protein: 60g. Fresh produce: tons of cucumbers, tomatoes, bell peppers, onions, and olives.

At the end of the day:

Skinny Woman ate a hot, guilt-free breakfast and a small, healthful lunch that (with the help of her later snack) allowed her to make it through the day without being exceedingly hungry. Dinner was her biggest meal, which was very satisfying after an entire day of strict self-control.

Calories: 860. That's *way* less than Skinny Woman's body burned—meaning her body will have to resort to burning excess FAT to get the extra energy it needs.

Protein: 87g. That's far more than the RDA, and it will totally help her body recover from all the exercise she's been getting lately, turning her flab into muscle.

Fresh produce: Every meal contained a substantial amount of vitamins, minerals, and fiber. What more could you ask for?

THE VERDICT

As I said, the results speak for themselves. Nevertheless, please allow me to summarize.

Skinny Woman consumed *fewer* calories, thereby causing her body to burn *more* of her fat reserves to make up for the missing calories, than did Average Woman. However, she also got *more* protein, *more* vitamins and minerals, *more* fiber, and *more* of the other essential nutrients than did Average Woman (who, by the way, did *NOT* eat *more* food).

THIS is why the "You mustn't eat fewer than 1200 calories per day" mantra is a MYTH. When you're trying to lose weight, it's the *nutrients*, not just the calories, that you need.

If you use the methods I recommend, tailored to your own body's particular needs, you will actually get way more essential nutrients in your diet than will the person who merely tries to "cut back" on her intake. You will be super healthy. You will get to eat several times throughout the day. You will enjoy healthful, satisfying meals. You will have a clear conscience when you consider what you're eating. You will have a healthy attitude towards food. You will be shedding excess fat faster than you ever did before, yet you will experience few—if any—adverse effects. You will be in little danger of starving yourself. You will feel like you are on top of the world. You will feel like a champion. You will *be* a champion! You may not have utilized the "right" methods, but you will have chosen the path that was right for you.

E | "I Don't Just Hate My Fat. Sometimes, I Hate Myself."

"I don't need to be better than others. I just want to be better than me."
- me, back in the beginning

Another thing that can kill your motivation is when you just don't like yourself very much. Why bother to change if you believe you're still going to be unhappy with the new you?

Just because this book is mostly upbeat doesn't mean that I don't know what it is to loathe myself. I know what it is to feel helpless, trapped in my body, to want to cut my fat off with a knife. I used to wonder if I might someday become one of those people who goes on disability pension and hides in their apartment because the world just seems too difficult to face. I get it.

The only way I have been able to lose weight is to be *positive* about it. And, importantly, to give thanks for everything I have. It hasn't all been natural for me, but I still tried, and the results speak for themselves.

I cry every time I look in the mirror.

Been there, done that. I have a story that might help.

I used to live in a really quiet neighborhood. A rather unclassy family moved into the house next door, and they brought *three* dogs with them. Loud outdoor dogs, naturally. Those bitches (haha) barked continually every morning, starting two hours before I wanted to wake up, and they made me *rage*. It got so bad, I found myself fantasizing about throwing poisoned food over the fence.

Eventually, because I couldn't change the fact that the dogs were there, I decided to try to change how I thought about the dogs. I started telling myself, *"Maybe those dogs aren't trying to ruin my morning; maybe they're just trying to be friendly! What if they're saying in doggie language, 'Hi! Hi! Hi there, neighbor, Hi! Hi!'?"* I conjured a silly image of goofy, friendly dogs wagging their tails. Soon, I found myself chuckling each time I heard them, and I was able to resume sleeping through their barking. All I had to do was reframe my thinking.

What does this story have to do with weight loss? I believe you can reframe the way you think when you're upset with your reflection. If you're anything like me, you're tempted to say *"F**k it! I try to lose weight and it doesn't work! I'm going to binge, baby, binge!"* Teach yourself instead to say, *"I worked hard yet didn't lose any weight? That can't go on forever; I'm going to keep trying—I know I MUST eventually see results!"* It has worked not only for me, but for many who suffer from the same pain and discouragement.

The girls I see in thinspo pictures are PERFECT. I want to look just like them, but I'm already skinny and don't look anything close.

Unfortunately, many of us CANNOT look like the gorgeous girls we see in pictures, because we simply have different genetic builds. Did you know, for example, that girls of Northern European lineage often have longer legs and higher buttocks than girls of Mediterranean European lineage do? Or that sub-Saharan Africans have larger butts and shorter, squatter calf muscles than others do? Or that East Asian women have less pronounced hourglass shapes than women elsewhere do? Even amongst local populations, there are huge variations in genetics and resulting body types.

You CAN achieve what is YOUR best body. However, if that's not what you had in mind when you started, you still won't like your body. If so, there's only one solution: you have to let it go. You did the best you could, and you ARE the best you can be. That alone is worth much. Moreover, getting to that place has probably made you far more beautiful on the inside, which is what counts—and it is what each of us will be left with in just a few more years of our bodies growing older.

I'm sorry this isn't as encouraging as you would like to hear. But you simply can't let yourself get caught up in thinking that you must look like a perfect version of *someone else*, rather than looking like the best version of *you*.

I'm afraid that once I lose the weight, I will still be ugly.

I sincerely doubt you are truly ugly. We all are our own worst critics, and we see ourselves in a much harsher light than others do. Still, even if you really, honestly can never look amazingly pretty … guess what? You still have to live your life. Being homely but healthy is a million times better than being fat is. Whether you have the genes of a "10" or the genes of a "1", you *will* look best at your healthiest weight.

Getting better-looking is only one of dozens of profoundly rewarding reasons to lose weight. Your life won't be perfect at a lower weight, but it will definitely be better. At the very least, you will know that you have succeeded in the battle against something that has triumphed over millions of others. Why wouldn't you want that?

Even when I reach my goal, I'll still have disgusting stretch marks. I'll never be happy and confident, and no-body will ever love me.

Although being fat is definitely enough to make one *unhappy*, you are correct that being thin won't make a person happy. Thin *gives* life, but it doesn't *fix* life.

Take a look around: although it seems that only the "beauti-ful people" are in love and happy, that's not true; they just hap-pen to be the ones we notice most. That's because they shine as our ideal, our fairly tale daydream.

However, you frequently see completely mismatched cou-ples all over the place. You know, the couples where one per-son is attractive and the other is surprisingly homely. Looking good is certainly not necessary. The couples who get together based on cuteness or hotness are the ones who split up after they start to take for granted the good looks that formerly had them so weak-kneed (hello, celebrity breakups!). Even if the relationship lasts well beyond that, many still often wind up di-vorced once their spouses' looks fade and they're left with what's inside. Love lasts when people love each other for who they *are*, not for how they look. Take comfort in that.

[NOTE: Much of this changes if you're in high school. High school isn't real life. Most schools should be torn down because they suck and needlessly torment millions of kids who would flourish but for the crappy environment. If you're forced to endure this evil in your life, just ride it out as best as you can, knowing that you will soon be able to enter the real world, where you will be free to be yourself.]

I'm just so tired of looking at everyone else being beautiful and having a good time. Why bother to live when I can't have that?

Satisfaction and fulfillment in life come not from what you look like, nor from who your friends are, nor from what you do. It comes from who you *are*. Being carried away by visions of being sexy and beautiful and popular is a common dream, yet it's little different from getting carried away by a destructive eating disorder. It's warm and glittery instead of dark and cold, but it's rooted in the same problem, namely, misplaced identity.

Nevertheless, let's indulge your fantasy for a moment. In your dream, you have a happy, carefree life where people adore you and approve of you. In reality, however, the problem is that they won't desire *you*, they will desire what you *have*, or in other words, what you do for *them*. The day will come, however, when you will no longer satisfy others' desires. What then? Then, you will be left with the You who is on the inside. That You will either be able to find contentment outside of others' approval, or it will completely fall apart without such approval. Like in so many things, the choices you make today will dictate how you wind up then.

How do you protect against this, regardless of what your life now looks like? You do it by choosing to invest in the long-term You instead of the fleeting you. Avoid comparing yourself to others, thereby sinking into an identity pit where, instead of being in control of your life and on top of the world, you become a slave to what others think of you. Rather, live the life of joy and freedom you envisioned. Go ahead and achieve your healthiest weight, and bask in the confidence it gives. Enjoy knowing that you are the best You that you can be. Nobody can take that from you, no matter what you (or they) look like in the end.

People say I'm not bad-looking, but I can't bring myself to believe them.

May I share a story? My life has long been marked by the same sentiment, and it took me until just recently to realize why.

Much of my upbringing involved emotional abuse. Like most kids, I didn't realize my life wasn't normal, and I just went along with it, never making the connection that it was actually the abuse that made me so critical of myself. At home, I was always told exactly what to do, and, usually, I didn't do it well enough. Even eating was like this: I ate what was put in front of me, but then I was later scolded for being fat. I was never encouraged to set goals and pursue them, I was only ever railed on for not living up to expectations.

No wonder I developed negative ideas about my identity, and no wonder it took me forever to figure out that I actually could succeed under my own initiative.

Years later, having lost a ton of weight and having become [what many people say is] good-looking, I still, on the inside, feel fairly ugly much of the time. Once, I even had a (gorgeous) guy who was interested in me, after he heard me mention something negative about myself, look me straight in the eye and say, "You're beautiful. I don't know why you're so down on yourself about your looks." All I could answer was that I guess that's just because I grew up without much approval at home. At the time, I really didn't realize how right I was.

Much later, I finally figured out what should have been obvious a long time ago, but for some reason I had remained blind to it: it *was* because of my upbringing that I was (and often am) so down on myself! In other words, when I'm tempted to feel worthless and unattractive, *it's not real!* It's just my twisted interpretation of things, warped by years of negative thinking.

Did you catch that? I'm going to say it one more time, so you take it to heart if it applies to you, too: often, when you think badly about yourself, it's not real, it's just how you see things at the moment. Much of the time when you're feeling condemned, unless you've actually done something to deserve condemnation, like going, "*Screw what's right, I'm choosing whatever I want, so Up Yours, World!*" your condemnation is misplaced.

The truth is, you have been given much. *You are beautiful and lovely in many ways, regardless of whether they are the types of beauty you would have chosen for yourself.* Celebrate and give thanks for those things, rather than focusing on the negatives.

If you can't stand your body, chances are, your body isn't the only problem (if it is even a problem at all). If you are beating yourself up over your behavior, you may actually be allowing someone else to beat you up. There's no need! Sometimes, just recognizing this can be a huge step toward victory.

F | Complaint Department (And, Is Big Beautiful?)

"Politically correct" is often only half true:
it always involves politics, but it's rarely correct.

PART ONE: THE COMPLAINT DEPARTMENT IS NOW OPEN

People often jump to the conclusion that I encourage anorexia because I sometimes embrace hunger and because I seek motivation in pictures of thin women. However, as you can surely see throughout this book, I actually advocate *healthy* eating. Besides, if pictures of skinny girls make people underweight, why does society get fatter and fatter the more access we have to fashion magazines and movies displaying slender people?

Anorexia rests more in the mind of the person than in her environment. It's rooted in self-hatred (to a degree) and in extreme perfectionism. It's often the fruit of a girl (or a guy, let's not forget) who feels like her eating is the only thing she can control in her out-of-control life. Well, guess what? Some of us are or were overweight because *we have self-control problems, too.* Yet, why don't others get as offended at restaurant commercials for bombarding us with food porn—showing gigantic portions of steaming food glistening with fat—as they get upset at thinspo for inspiring girls to seek a healthy weight by reminding them of what they can achieve? The level of hypocrisy is remarkable.

People are unfair to underweight girls. Underweight girls reliably get as much or more hate than even the fattest of people. Yet obesity can be as much a mental disorder as anorexia is—how else can you account for someone being unable to stop doing something (overeating) which is killing them? Why, then, are underweight people reviled while fat people remain relatively unscathed? Probably because few envy fat people.

Anorexia is horrible. Obesity is horrible. *There's no easy an-*

swer to this.

How the hell does thin *"give life"?*

Get fat, and you'll quickly figure it out.

Being thin won't make a person happy.

Correct. However, being thin gives freedom from the debilitating misery and depression (and health detriments) that accompany fatness. *That* gives happiness.

You're helping people to live a wrong lifestyle.

I'm trying to help people to *flee*, like I fled, a "wrong lifestyle" of eating far more than we need and suffering the misery that comes with it. I merely echo what our physicians keep telling us: eat less than we have been eating, exercise more than we currently do.

The *other* wrong lifestyle, the eating disordered lifestyle, is something I try to *discourage*. I tell nobody to stop eating. I caution against fasting as a weight loss method. I never tell anyone that they shouldn't be happy until they are perfect—nor that obtaining perfection will make them happy. On the contrary, I actually cheer and applaud everyone who tries to avoid becoming overly skinny.

This book doesn't trap unwary girls, happy with their weights, and sell them into slavery to an eating disorder. It is merely a help to those who find inspiration, encouragement, and comfort within its pages. All I seek is to celebrate beauty, to share what works for me, and to allow others to take courage in knowing that they are not nearly as alone as they felt before.

You're still wrong. You encourage anorexia. My friend used to be obsessed with dieting and purging. People like you make her miserable.

I don't encourage anorexia; I encourage skinny. There's a difference. *Anorexia* means obsessing over food and not eating enough of it. *Skinny* means making mature choices to get your body back to its healthiest and most attractive weight.

Yes, I'm sad that some people let their dieting get out of

control. It's perplexing, however, to see that some are more concerned about the unhappiness of those who take their dieting too far than they are about the shame and misery that fat people must daily endure when they can't shake their excess weight. Each of us has our own demons to fight.

I'm not saying that this is the only way. I'm saying it's the only way *for some of us*, the only *effective* way for us to heal. For some of us who have tried everything else and failed, and who have wondered time and time again if we must simply always be fat, this is what works. This is what strengthens us to make healthy decisions and to take control of our lives.

But it's wrong to want to be skinny.

If the desire is so uncontrollable that it causes an ED, then yes, it's a problem. But let's also look at the problem of when a person doesn't desire skinny *enough*.

Doing a little online research, I found that being overweight or obese is America's second leading cause of death. Yet anorexia is responsible for only about 0.01% of American women's deaths. Furthermore, about 30% of American teens are overweight, and another 15% are obese. That's a total of 45% who need to lose weight! In the same population, guess how many are anorexic. That's right, 1%. We have a 45:1 ratio of too-fat to too-skinny teens.

So if it's wrong to be overweight and wrong to be underweight, why is it overwhelmingly the experience of the skinny people that they are the ones constantly harassed about their eating? How much more often are skinny kids told to eat than fat kids are told to put the donut down? How can this be objective, rooted in concern for the person's health, and not rooted merely in envy?

Consider the following things commonly heard by people on various places along the weight spectrum when they mention that they are watching what they eat:

- *Obese person:* "It's hard being healthy in our society … here, have a donut."
- *Overweight person:* "No big deal, honey, we all want to lose a few pounds."
- *Healthy / thin person:* "So that's how you do it! I wish I had your self-control."

- *But the second someone crosses into the "Underweight" range:* "What's wrong with you, anorexic freak? That's it, we're locking you up until you get fatter! You're just vain!"

You know it's true.

Please give the skinny girls a break.

Fat people are people, too!

Yes, I know, *I used to be one!* I also know that fat people often *loathe* their fat and feel *trapped* in their bodies. Fat people know they're just as clever and lovely and worthy on the inside as other people are. Yet, tragically, when others judge fat people by their appearance, the next thing you know, the fat people are judging themselves the same way.

Yes, it sucks to be a fat person. But the good news is, we *don't* have to stay fat!

You don't really think everyone judges by looks, do you?

I was fat all my life and sometimes still feel like I am. That lifetime of experience, and now my experience on the other side, reveals that the world really does judge us by our looks. Don't believe me? Try going into a nice store dressed in your gym clothes. Then come back a few weeks later dressed in your best clothing with your hair and makeup perfect, and compare the level of respect you get.

You judge by appearances, too, in ways you probably don't even realize, and which may have nothing to do with fat or skinny. If you think you don't instinctively judge by appearances, or at least are not tempted to, you're being dishonest with yourself.

Being fat erects a barrier between fat people and the rest of the world. Often, other people eventually surmount this barrier and come to know and love the person inside, but it takes time for them to get past their prejudices. Seriously, even fat people judge other fat people for being fat. Or for being too skinny. Or for almost anything, even for being too good-looking. Have you never seen a gorgeous girl and thought, "*She must be so shallow and full of herself.*"?

We must come to terms with the fact that the world is the way it is, not the way we wish it was. If being fat puts up an unnecessary barrier between someone and others, it make sense to remove that barrier—by dealing with the fat.

It's wrong to use pictures of thin girls to motivate you to lose weight.

This makes my heart sink. If only you could see all the tears I cried over the years, all the self-condemnation I endured, thinking I was always and only ever going to be a fat loser, because I could never find the inspiration to do what it takes to lose weight.

That was until I found thinspo. Thinspo reminded me that everyone has the potential to be slender and beautiful. It reminded me of how far I had to go, but it gave me the hope of a wonderful reward when I arrived. It sparked a fire in me and fueled my passion for healthy eating and healthy living.

Now, later, I stand a testament to the power of thinspo. I lost a ton of weight. I got fit. I ceased to be an ugly duckling and embraced my inner swan. I ceased to resent who I was and became grateful for who I am. I ceased frowning on the inside and started wearing a daily smile. I changed forever. I found new life.

Furthermore, I learned to be *inspired* by others' success instead of resenting them for it. I learned that I can also inspire others. I learned that I don't have to be a prisoner to my desires. I learned that I can be happy with my body instead of ashamed of it. I learned that it's possible to introduce myself to people without first feeling like I have to apologize for being a failure. I learned that it's possible to do this, and to do it safely, without developing an ED. I learned that even though there are some of us out there who have lived for years tempted to feel like we are worthless, and have come to accept that "fact" as a deep-rooted and debilitating facet of our identity ... we aren't worthless after all. I learned that we can emerge from our comas of crippling self-hatred and embarrassing lack of self-control and become the people we were meant to be.

If thinspo can do that, bring it on.

All bodies are beautiful no matter how much they weigh.

Ah, the "fat positive" or "fat acceptance" movement.

Realizing that many people are really down on themselves

because they're fat, a group decided to spread the idea that fat is just as beautiful as thin, and that anyone who disagrees is merely brainwashed. Let's assume for the sake of argument that the people who started this weren't bitter about their own looks but meant well and merely desired to spread positivity around the world.

The problem is, I've checked out the "fat positive" websites. The girls there really don't seem positive at all. In fact, the attitude I found was a total downer; it seemed false and even a bit creepy. You've got these *obviously* overweight and even obese people saying, "I love my fat body!" Many of them even qualify themselves by mentioning how hard it is to believe it when they say it. It really seems like an unhealthy delusion, like the heavy counterpart to anorexic girls who believe they're fat and try to confess that they're thin but can't bring themselves to do it.

The sad fact is, fat is a sign of poor health and poor self-control. What's positive about that?

I know that this response might hurt feelings. At the same time, I believe that pain is sometime the best motivator. Is it worse to hurt someone by telling them the truth or to hurt them by lying to them and letting them self-destruct? Think about it. Are we next to tell addicts to keep doing drugs, alcoholics to have another drink, and cutters to push the blade a little deeper? That's what logically follows once you abandon reason—as many of the fat acceptance proponents seem to have done.

There is way too much self-hate out there. I get it when people say we should be happy with our bodies. When our bodies are at a medically healthy weight, that makes sense. The problem I have is not with people who genuinely worry that some girls are too hard on themselves, but with those who feed girls lies in an attempt to heal them, and who then jump all over you when you point out the lie. Someone needs to tell those people that The Emperor is Naked.

PART TWO: IS BIG BEAUTIFUL?

You've heard it a million times, so it must be true: modern society is screwed up and has departed from the sensible days of old when full-figured women were considered the most attractive … right?

Proponents of this philosophy work tirelessly to find facts to support their claims. Sometimes, they don't even bother supporting their claims, but merely assert that things should be obvious from looking at the "evidence". However, evidence can often support multiple theories. When the theories oppose each other, only one can be correct. Keeping this in mind, let's examine the arguments.

Paintings and sculptures of women from centuries ago consist of plump women with rolls, proving that such women were the ideal, and had the look that really captured the gents' attention back in the day.

Question: do you realize that people who have never been to the USA think young Americans do nothing but party and have sex all the time? We have "reality TV" to thank for this. Similarly, many Americans who haven't been to California think it's all palm trees, beaches, and beautiful people (or that Los Angeles is just one big gun battle). When producers get to edit every shot for their TV shows, they can make it look like that—but the truth is, most of California and its citizenry looks like anywhere else.

Similarly, you can't form an impression about a society based on a handful of art productions. Art *imitates* life, but does not necessarily *depict* life. Artists often reside on the fringes of society, and hang out with a unique crowd. It has always been so. We cannot necessarily rely on artistic works as representing the *mainstream* culture of the day.

Then there's The Louvre. Yes, of course, the Louvre displays statue after statue and wall after wall of paintings depicting roly-poly courtesans in carefree repose. But you know what else? The entire museum is *crammed* with sexual content. Wing upon wing of the museum is pornographic. It makes one feel dirty being in the midst of it all. Couldn't these artists find *any*-

thing more normal to portray than such sultry and scandalous subjects? The artwork in question can hardly be representative of life as seen by the average, everyday, church-going person of the era.

One must also inquire: where did the artists find their models? They would have needed models to sit topless for days. Who do you think had the *time* to sit around posing for sculptors? Was it regular women with responsibilities like cooking, cleaning, and surviving the tough times they faced centuries ago? Or was it portly princesses and duchesses-to-be with plenty of leisure time to hang out with their artist friends?

Furthermore, art history itself throws a wrench into the gears of this argument. There exist thousands of examples of artwork, from across the millennia, depicting the glory of the female body in a slender, toned and even bony form. Their sculptors and painters were *contemporaries* of the artists who preferred their muses portly. Many ancient Greek and Roman statues depict perfectly thinspo-worthy babes, complete with abs, hipbones, toned arms, tiny bottoms, and pointy shoulderblades. Even many Renaissance paintings show similarly slender women—not always very toned women (I guess in the 1500s you worked with whomever you could convince to get naked), but certainly lacking in rolls or double chins.

Finally, why is it only the *artists* you hear referenced in support of this "big was beautiful" theory? Where are the *historians* who wrote about what the ladies aspired to look like? What about literature from writers in foreign cultures who coveted the physiques of these Plump Ladies of Paris? Can't *anyone* produce the diary of some forlorn thin girl who just wished she could become a size XL?

None of it adds up. So please don't believe it. Apparently, for a short time, a few painters and sculptors pulled out their tools in the presence of some girls who lived really easy lives. They are the exception, not the rule, in the history of human beauty.

In feudal times, only peasants were slender, and the rich were plump. Being skinny meant you were poor. Nobody found such women attractive.

Seriously? *When* has social class *ever* been a factor in deciding which women are attractive? Although women frequently will disregard a man's looks if he's rich, famous, powerful, or otherwise successful, none of these things usually factors into a woman's attractiveness. For women, hot has always been hot. What homely girl dreams of becoming rich, famous, or powerful in order to find her dream mate? Rather, she dreams of becoming *beautiful*.

In the ancient story of Esther, for example, the king chose the prettiest girl—even though she was a commoner who belonged to a locally-despised minority—to become his queen. Similarly, other tales from time immemorial are rife with stories of princes and other high-status men falling for pretty servant girls. Sure, some such works are fiction—but they're far less fanciful than the claim that nobody used to find thin girls attractive.

Eating disorders are a modern phenomenon, and are the fruit of a screwed-up culture obsessed with thin.

One of the most important maxims in research is that *correlation does not imply causation*. Things can have a pattern of occurring together, but that does *not* mean that one causes the other. For example, some used to think that living under power wires caused health problems, because people whose homes were under the wires had more health issues. It must be the electromagnetic radiation emanating from the wires that causes health problems, right? Actually, no. It turns out that the ugliness of the power wires lowered the values of the homes situated under them, and only the poorest people—those who often have a harder time maintaining good diet, health and hygiene practices—would choose to live there.

So it is, I believe, with EDs. The number of reported cases of EDs is growing. However, that's just *reported cases*. Does that mean that EDs were never occurring before? It can just as easily mean they were simply going undiagnosed.

There's more. Did you know that the *number* of EDs that psychologists test for has also increased? There used to be only anorexia and bulimia. If you were *really* close to having either disorder, but just didn't quite make it because you lacked just one of the required symptoms—or if you exhibited all the symptoms but just not quite strongly enough—you didn't officially have an eating disorder. Then they added EDNOS ("Eating Disorder Not Otherwise Specified"), and suddenly, all these "almost there but not quite" people now "had" EDs, because there then existed a classifiable ED to match their lesser symptoms. It doesn't end there, either. Guess what? They just added another, Binge Eating Disorder, and they made other disorders easier to find in a person, for example by removing the anorexia requirements that the person be drastically underweight or that they fear gaining weight. Hello, sudden increase in ED diagnoses!

Psychology, as a science, is barely over a century old. It is still in its infancy compared to Medicine and the other sciences. There's no way there won't be more and more "disorders" discovered (meaning, somebody in a white coat gives a certain behavior a name) as time goes on, bringing a corresponding "alarming increase" in the number who suffer from mental disorders.

Let's pull all this together. Let's assume that "media and social pressure" to be thin really is on the rise. That still doesn't mean it is *causing* the prevalence of EDs to rise. Cutting and other forms of self-harm are also *really* on the rise. Do we blame *that* on pressure for girls to be thin? You almost have to, because almost all the media and social pressure out there is for girls *not* to harm themselves, so that's obviously not what's causing them to cut. EDs stem from a wrong view of self—just like cutting does—and should not be blamed on a society that just happens to notice that thin can be beautiful.

Too many girls hate themselves as it is. Here's a concept: *how about we divert the energy spent passing judgment* on people who admire slender physiques, and *instead spend that energy showing the self-harming girls that they are loved?*

That's what I intend to do.

In remote, isolated cultures that formerly had little access to Western media, nobody used to have EDs. Now that these cultures have internet, TV, and Western fashion influences, EDs are cropping up all over the place.

True enough. And also on the rise is every other ill that Western society suffers, *especially* obesity! Correlation does not imply causation. Let's move on.

It's only because of the evil fashion industry and media that women today want to be thin.

We all can tell that the fashion industry is not run by normal-thinking people, and that the media merely parrot what the fashion industry comes up with. Finding examples is easy. Go online and click around a social media website where people share pictures of pretty girls. Something like a "real girl thinspo" site, or a site devoted to beauty, or some such thing (but not a pro-ana site or a fashion site). You will see page after page of elegant, girly prettiness and beachy cuteness, almost all of which is at a healthy weight. *This* is what *normal* people find beautiful enough to post on internet pages, and it's what normal people aspire to.

Next, look up pictures of the world's top 100 female fashion models. There's a handful of babes in there, but many of the rest are a little odd-looking. Instead of being girly, they tend to have the facial features (and often the bodily shape) of gangly and awkward adolescent boys. I'm not making this up, and I'm not being unkind. People have studied it and written about it. Seriously, look with an open mind, and you'll see it.

Now, ask yourself how much sense it makes to think that most people, who when left to their own devices gravitate toward girly beauty, would allow fashion magazines to influence them so much that they think, "*Screw my gut instinct, freaky is beautiful!*" You're not that stupid, so please don't tolerate others' saying you are.

Even if you set aside the actual features of the models and focus purely on their skinniness, there's still no reason to blame the fashion industry for society's preference for skinny. Those magazines are there for ONE reason only: to SELL. If people were drawn to plumper models, they would buy the magazines filled with big butts and heaving bosoms. Such magazine exist, but they are rarely the ones that sell.

Psychological tests prove that people find curvy women, even a little overweight, the most attractive.

The tests you refer to are the "line drawing" and "silhouette" tests where they show a row of female figures, thin on one side, and increasing in fatness until you get to the other side. These are not real photographs of real women showing their actual features. They're synthetic, designed to eliminate other factors of beauty. Testers ask people to rate the most attractive figures, which often seem to wind up having a slightly higher BMI than people would choose were they rating pictures of actual women.

This trying to prove that plumper silhouettes are most attractive is flawed. You can't tell how attractive someone is from just her profile. The taut tummy, the slight ripple of ribs, the defined collarbones, the lines, contours, and shadows cast by various muscles and bones, and all the other delicate and feminine features that *appear only in slender women* are LOST when using generic profiles. Literally all that the researchers have proven with these tests is that in the absence of other visible features, curvy hips and hourglass figures look good on women.

However, this does *not* prove that fat looks good or that skinny looks bad. There are women out there with almost no fat on their bodies who have incredible bone structure, giving them broad shoulders, wide hips, and narrow waists. Likewise, there are heavier women with boxier shapes. You know which shape is going to turn heads.

Marilyn Monroe was considered sexy in her day, yet she would be considered too fat for Hollywood today.

Why is Marilyn Monroe the ONLY actress we typically hear brought up in this argument? If super-curvy women were all the rage back then, why was only ONE such woman considered sexy? Where is the list of similarly heavy stars? No such list exists.

Seriously, just look at a small sample of the top leading ladies of film from the days of old: Grace Kelly. Katharine Hepburn. Ingrid Bergman. Bette Davis. Greta Garbo. Joan Crawford. Lauren Bacall. Vivian Leigh. Sophia Loren. A person could rattle off names all day. The point is, not ONE of these women was anything but slender and elegant. There's not a heavy woman among them. But they were always considered the embodiment of beautiful. Look them up yourselves. All you see are defined jaws, prominent collarbones, and narrow waists.

So what made Marilyn Monroe so popular?[22] She had a cute

---

[22] Be sure to remember: when she *first* came onto the scene, Marilyn Monroe *was* rather tiny. She became more full-figured *after* she had obtained a reputation for hotness..

face, sure, but what was she *really* known for? For displaying herself in Playboy (as you can imagine, the first centerfold of the first mainstream porn magazine is obviously going to cause quite a stir), for taking seductress roles in movies, for having something suspicious going on with (married) President Kennedy, and for living a generally promiscuous life. Of course she's going to get a following of heavy-breathing MEN. What man isn't going to take notice of a big-chested blonde who likes to tease? This seems like a pretty sensible reason why Marilyn Monroe had a reputation for being "sexy".

But consider this: what other actress in Marilyn Monroe's time was making waves with her stunning beauty? Which actress did the *women* (and, I imagine, the classier men) admire? Who did the *women* wish they could be like? That's right, Audrey Hepburn. Audrey Hepburn, perhaps the most remarkably slender woman ever to star in film. Audrey Hepburn, whose pictures appeared on every mainstream magazine's cover, and whose image still sells today. Where did Marilyn Monroe's pictures appear? On the walls of mechanics' garages and hidden beneath teenaged boys' mattresses.

In an online search of each actress, reading only the first three lines of text, I found the following: Audrey Hepburn, a "film and fashion icon" who "redefined glamour." Marilyn Monroe, a "sex symbol." Need I really say any more?

Fine, then. Why don't you tell me why the focus on thin has grown so much in recent history?

Think on this: before the second half of the 20th Century, there was no such thing as low-rider jeans, short skirts (or short shorts), tank tops, two-piece bathing suits, or even fitted T-shirts. Women wore dresses, or perhaps knee-length skirts with blouses (even the name "blouse" implies that the garment blouses out and away from the body). They buttoned up their collars. They certainly showed little skin beyond the occasional knee or elbow.

In a setting like that, what kinds of things would make people stop and stare when a woman walked by? Opportunities to show off a tight butt, flat stomach, pokey hipbones, and all those things we love about thinspo—they simply didn't exist. The only things that really stood out as indicators of femininity were pretty faces, big chests, and wide hips. That's it. How else would corsets have become popular if not because they exaggerated the chest, hips, and—oh yeah—a small waist. Years ago, you simply had fewer reasons to work on getting skinny, because you and your husband were the only ones who would notice the results.

Today, however, most garments cling tightly to your body, and show off every imperfection—as well as every part you worked so hard to make slender and beautiful. When did attire like this start coming around? The bikini was introduced in the 1940s, miniskirts in the 60s, skintight jeans in the 70s, crop tops took off in the 90s ... and now we have yoga pants.

The only way "society has changed" is to permit skimpier and skimpier outfits revealing more and more feminine beauty, thereby giving women a greater incentive to work on perfecting their bodies. Is this wrong? Possibly. But being skinny is not.

ONE LAST THOUGHT

In closing, consider this: have you ever heard the expression, "I need to watch what I eat, because I don't want to lose my womanly figure"? Didn't think so. It's a *girlish* figure—that is, a *slender* figure—that women have wanted since time began. It's not rocket science.

Can you be overweight and beautiful? Of course you can. But this battle cry of "*It's all modern society's fault that you want to be thin*" distorts history. Its proponents would do well to give us all a little credit for being able to make up our own minds about what look we like best.

Last Word | Is Skinny a Valid Goal, Revisited

As of this writing, my weight is a handful of pounds over my original Goal Weight. It's a healthy weight, and it looks alright on me, it's just not exactly thinspo weight. I jiggle more when I run, and my jeans aren't nearly as roomy as I would like them to be. But I know that nobody who meets me thinks of me as fat, nor do they ever suspect that I once was.

I also know that I was happier and more confident when I was thinner, and I want to get back to that place. It will be a hard road for me to get there, but it will be worth it when I arrive (and I promise you, I *will* arrive—and I'm already back on my way down).

Yet, at the same time, I know I can give too much weight (pun not intended) to the importance of being skinny. Like I once wrote, I need not just my body but also my mind and heart to be light.

Right now, I'm healthy, I look decent, and I am fairly fit. Some people tell me I look better at this weight than I did when I was at my skinniest. I believe they are sincere, and I understand what they mean.

But, obviously, I disagree, and it's frustrating: I don't want to be just alright, I want to be *gorgeous*. I want to be *amazing*. I want to be *perfect*.

Yet, I also don't want infatuation with perfection to consume me. Any of us, if we're not careful, can become just another number, another casualty in the weight loss war. That war has already claimed too many. Life is too short to allow ourselves to become miserable over such an unimportant thing as a little extra padding. Strangers' opinions matter too little to allow ourselves to worry about how attractive others find us.

When I examine myself without letting emotions get in the way, I realize this: I lost weight, I found life, and I became the person I never thought I could be. I should be happy. I *am* happy whenever I don't allow negative thoughts, self-criticism, and an unrealistic desire for perfection to overcome common sense.

Would I like to lose a little more fat, to reach what I believe is my "best" weight? Yes. Will I feel like a failure if I don't? My instinct is to say Yes, but if I'm honest, the answer is No. I'm not a failure. *I'm not a failure!* I am who I am on the inside, and on the outside I'm no longer handicapped by that fat person with whom I used to identify. I should be content with that. It is enough.

I know that "thin gives life." I've personally experienced some of the best life that thin can give. It's just not that thin *is* life.

So it's time for me to move on. It's time to explore those other important things which make for a joyful and successful life, and to not remain stuck dwelling on my weight. In the meantime, I'll always be keeping an eye on my weight, always recording it on a graph next to my bathroom scale, always struggling to find the balance between enjoying food and fearing it. But that's just being human. It's normal. It's called life.

And it's just lovely to be alive.

To Be Continued …

(In my life and in yours)

About the Author

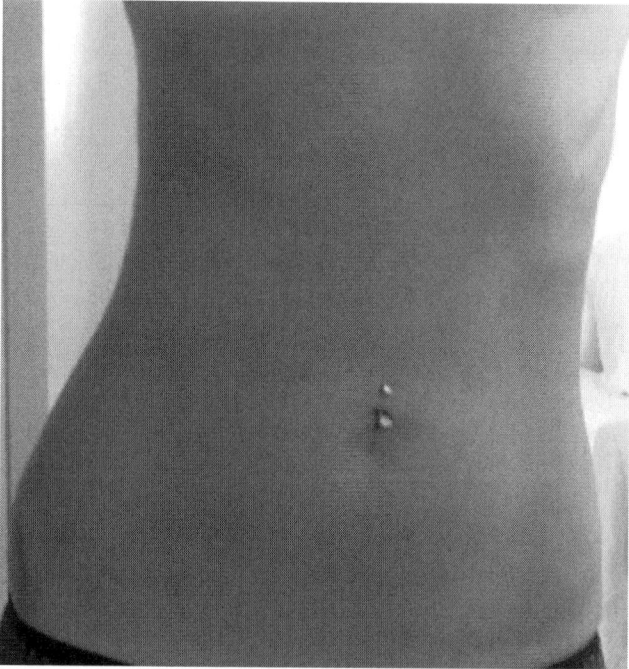

Alyssa Dahl lives happily and healthily in California and enjoys a career in an area unrelated to health and fitness. She prefers to stay out of the spotlight, and both apologizes for this and appreciates others' willingness to grant her that courtesy.

None of this matters, of course, as this book is about you, not her. So get out there, become your best, and never look back.

Further Reading & Contact Information

For information about this book or its author, or to find out where you can find vast amounts of beautiful thinspo, visit:

therealyouisskinny.wordpress.com
sweetthinspiration.tumblr.com
twitter: @AlyssaMDahl

Medical and mental health professionals are encouraged to distribute certain portions of this work free of charge. Please see the copyright page for details.

Copies of this book are also available, at cost, for clinical use. For details, please contact the author at the above website(s).

To others who would like free or at-cost copies of this book, please contact the author, who is always looking to support a good cause.

Printed in Great Britain
by Amazon

62166830R00165